Pediatric Cardiology for the House Officer

BOOKS IN THE HOUSE OFFICER SERIES

Burn Care for the House Officer

Cardiology for the House Officer, Second Edition

Clinical Pathology for the House Officer

Critical Care Medicine for the House Officer

Dermatology for the House Officer, Second Edition

Diabetes Mellitus for the House Officer

Diagnostic Radiology for the House Officer

Emergency Medicine for the House Officer

Emergency Psychiatry for the House Officer

Endocrinology for the House Officer

Hematology for the House Officer, Second Edition

Infectious Disease for the House Officer

Neurology for the House Officer, Third Edition

Neurosurgical Management for the House Officer

Obstetrics for the House Officer

Pediatric Cardiology for the House Officer

Pediatric Neurology for the House Officer, Second Edition

Psychiatry for the House Officer, Second Edition

Respiratory Medicine for the House Officer, Second Edition

Therapeutic Radiology for the House Officer

Vascular Surgery for the House Officer

BOOKS IN THE CASE STUDIES FOR THE HOUSE OFFICER SERIES

Case Studies in Cardiology for the House Officer

Case Studies in Endocrinology for the House Officer

Case Studies in Neurology for the House Officer

Case Studies in Neurosurgery for the House Officer

Case Studies in Psychiatry for the House Officer

Pediatric Cardiology for the House Officer

Edmond J. Sacks, M.D., F.A.A.P., F.A.C.C.
Director, Pediatric Cardiology
Jefferson Medical College
Thomas Jefferson University
Philadelphia, Pennsylvania

WILLIAMS & WILKINS
Baltimore • London • Los Angeles • Sydney

Editor: Nancy Collins
Associate Editor: Carol Eckhart
Copy Editor:
Design: JoAnne Janowiak
Illustration Planning: Wayne Hubbel
Production: Raymond E. Reter

Accurate indications, adverse reactions, and dosage schedules for drugs are provided in this book, but it is possible that they may change. The reader is urged to review the package information date of the manufacturers of the medications mentioned.

Printed in the United States of America

Library of Congress Cataloging in Publication Data

Sacks, Edmond J.
Pediatric cardiology for the house officer.
(The House office series)
Includes bibliographies and index.
1. Pediatric cardiology. I. Title. II. Series. [DNLM: 1. Cardiovascular Diseases—in infancy & childhood. WS 290 S121p]
RJ421.S23 1987 618.92′12 86-28210
ISBN 0-683-07487-3

86 87 88 89 90 10 9 8 7 6 5 4 3 2 1

TO ELLEN, GABRIELL, AND JOSH

TO FLORENCE AND HERMAN

TO DRS. ABE RUDOLPH, JULIEN HOFFMAN, MICHAEL HEYMANN, PAUL STANGER, DON RITTER, AND ALEX NADAS FOR ILLUMINATING PEDIATRIC CARDIOLOGY

Preface

Because pediatric cardiology is one of the newer subspecialties, it is common to wonder what problems generally involve the pediatric cardiologist. The historical beginnings of pediatric cardiology largely involved detection, diagnosis, and management of congenital heart disease, as well as acute rheumatic fever. Although acute rheumatic fever is now rare, involvement with congenital heart disease persists today. However, pediatric cardiology now has a much broader base which includes sophisticated analysis (electrophysiological studies) and management of pediatric cardiac dysrhythmias, creative, advanced palliative and corrective surgical techniques, interventional cardiac catheterization techniques, as well as preventive pediatric cardiology. The purpose of this book is to present a concise overview of major areas of pediatric cardiology with emphasis upon accurate detection and diagnosis, followed by logical management. Because of space limitations, in-depth discussion of many topics will not be possible; however, pertinent references will guide the reader to further elaboration of these subjects. Where possible, tables, analogy, and outline will replace lengthy text to allow the reader to focus upon important points and concepts. New tables of ECG normal values, a new diagrammatic format to represent individual congenital cardiac defects, and a brief discussion of ethical issues are included. For the author, it has been a privilege to practice pediatric cardiology during an era of such great diagnostic and surgical advances, as well as during the development of interventional catheterization.

Preface

Contents

Chapter 1

Hereditable Aspects of Pediatric Cardiology

The incidence of congenital heart disease [CHD] has remained rather constant over the past several decades in most populations across the world. Eight to ten per one thousand [8-10/ 1,000] liveborn infants, will have a congenital cardiac malformation. Distribution of the five most common defects depends upon age at presentation, per Table 1.1. To explain recurrence rates of CHD, one must use concepts of multifactorial inheritance, which involves an interaction between genetic propensity and the environment. Based upon previous experience, the risk of a child being born with CHD in a given family with no previous CHD would be approximately 0.8 - 1.0% [8-10/1,000 liveborn]. Suggested risks of recurrence in families with one parent or with one sibling who has one of the more common forms of CHD are listed in Table 1.3, and are in the range of 1-4%. If one considers all possible congenital malformations of the heart, the usual recurrence figure is 5% if a family has one affected first degree relative. This figure must be tempered by recent data from Toronto, Canada, that suggests recurrence rates may vary according to the population studied. This study reported an incidence as high as 10% in offspring of 219 parents [only one parent had a cardiac defect in any family] with either atrial septal defect, aortic coarctation, aortic stenosis, or complex dextrocardia. Recurrence risk decreased to 8.8% if one excluded mitral valve prolapse and Wolff-Parkinson-White syndrome. The authors attribute this increased incidence to environmental rather than genetic factors (1). Another very recent study suggests recurrence rates for aortic coarctation and for hypoplastic left heart syndrome may be as high as 8% and 12-14% respectively, when there is one affected sibling in an index family. This epidemiologic study further divided congenital cardiac defects into pathogenic groups of abnormal: [1] tissue migration, [2] blood flow, [3] cell death, [4] extracellular matrix, [5] targeted growth. Study results indicate that left heart blood flow defects have a higher recurrence rate than previously noted (2). These new data appear in parentheses in Table 1.3. In families having two affected first degree relatives with CHD, risk triples to approximately 12-15%. In the unusual family with more than two affected first degree relatives, risk could become greater than Mendelian autosomal dominant traits, or greater than 50%.

Although not consistently associated with CHD, there are certain medications, maternal illnesses, and other agents that result in a higher than usual incidence of congenital cardiac defects. These associations are listed in Table 1.2. Although not hereditable in the usual sense, CHD is associated with many hereditable disorders as outlined in Table 1.4. Note that certain lesions such as hypertrophic obstructive cardiomyopathy are transmitted as a dominant trait with variable penetrance [see Chapter 9]. Rarely there is familial clustering of atrial septal defect, forms of tetralogy of Fallot, and first degree A-V Block. A very rare dominant pattern of hereditability has recently been reported for aortic coarctation and many investigators consider mitral valve prolapse hereditary.

Other Familial Cardiovascular Associations in Pediatric Patients: In addition to possible familial occurrence of congenital heart disease, studies now demonstrate family clustering of the following cardiovascular problems:

[1] Hypertension/ [2] Cardiac Dysrhythmias/
[3] Hyperlipoproteinemias/ [4] Panic Attack Syndrome

Table 1.1: Five Most Common Congenital Cardiac Defects Relative to Age at Presentation (3)

AGE [DAYS]: RANK	0-6 [%]	7-13 [%]	13-20 [%]	180-365 [%]
1	TGV [17]	AC [19]	VSD [20]	VSD [20]
2	HLHS [12]	VSD [15]	TGV [17]	PDA/TOF [14]
3	TOF [9]	HLHS [11]	AC [16]	ASD [10]
4	AC/ VSD/ PA/IVS [7]	TGV [9]	TOF [8]	ECD/MYO [7]
5	HETERO [6]	TOF [6]	ECD/ HETERO [6]	PS [6]

KEY:
AC: Aortic Coarctation
AS: Aortic Stenosis
ASD: Atrial Septal Defect
ECD: Endocardial Cushion Defects
HETERO: Heterotaxias
HLHS: Hypoplastic Left Heart Syndrome

MYO: Myocardial Disease
PA/IVS: Pulmonary Atresia with Intact Ventricular Septum
PDA: Patent Ductus Arteriosus
PS: Pulmonary Stenosis
TGV: Complete Transposition of the Great Vessels (D-Loop,D-Transposition/ Cyanotic Newborn)
TOF: Tetralogy of Fallot (Large VSD with PS)
VSD: Ventricular Septal Defect

Table 1.2: Maternal Infection, Illness, or Medication Associated with a Higher than Usual Incidence of Congenital Heart Disease (4)

Agent/Illness	% Effected by exposure	Associations
Alcohol	25-30	VSD/PDA/ASD
Amphetamines	5 (?)	VSD/PDA/ASD/TGV
Hydantoin	2- 3	PS/AS/AC/PDA
Trimethadione	15-30	TGV/TOF/HLHS
Chemotherapy	5 (?)	PS/AS/VSD/ASD
Lithium	10	Ebstein/TA/ASD
Reproductive Hormones [A]	2- 4	VSD/TGV/TOF
Thalidomide	5-10	TOF/VSD/ASD/ Truncus
Rubella	35	PPS/PDA/VSD/ASD
Diabetes	3- 5	TGV/VSD/AC
	30-50	Cardiomegaly/ Cardiomyopathy
Lupus Erythematosis	(?)	Complete Heart Block
Phenylketonuria	25-50	TOF/VSD/ASD

Key: Per Table 1.1/ Truncus=Truncus Arteriosus/ PPS=Peripheral Pulmonary Stenosis/ TA= Tricuspid Atresia

[A] Recent evidence indicates that there is no higher incidence of malformations in offspring of mothers exposed to reproductive hormones. These important studies suggest that it may be necessary to re-evaluate many previous correlations between agents taken during gestation and their possible teratogenicity (5,6).

Table 1.3: Recurrence Rate for Specific Congenital Cardiac Abnormalities if One Parent or Sibling Has a Congenital Heart Defect (7)

DEFECT	Suggested Recurrence Risk with One Parent [%]/	with One Sibling [%]
VSD	4	3
PDA	4	3
ASD	2.5	2.5
TOF	4	2.5
PS	3.5	2
AC	2	2 [8] (8)
AS	4	2
TGV		2
A-V Canal		2
EFE		4
TA		1
Ebstein		1
Truncus Arteriosus		1
Pulmonary Atresia		1
HLHS		2 [12-14] (9)

KEY: Per Tables 1.1/1.2: EFE=Endocardial Fibroelastosis

Table 1.4: Hereditable Disorders Associated with Cardiac Disease (10)

Chromosomal and Miscellaneous Abnormalities:

Disorder	% Incidence of CHD	Associations
GENERAL POPULATION	1	VSD/ PDA/ ASD
Trisomy 21 [Down]	50	VSD/ ECD/ ASD/ PDA
Trisomy 22	65	ASD/ VSD
Trisomy 13	90	VSD/ PDA/ Dextro-version
Trisomy 18	99+	VSD/ PDA/ PS
4p-	40	VSD/ ASD/ PDA
5p- [Cri-du-Chat]	25	VSD/ PDA/ ASD
13q-	50	VSD
18q-	50	VSD
C Group Anomalies	25-50	VSD/ PDA
XO [Turner]	35	AC/ AS/ ASD
XXXXY	14	PDA/ ASD

DiGeorge Syndrome	>85	Conotruncal abnormalities/ VSD/aortic atresia

RECESSIVE SYNDROMES:

Adrenogenital [21/3]	Hyperkalemia/ Broad QRS/ Arrhythmias
Alkaptonuria	Atherosclerosis/ Valve Disease
Carpenter	PDA
Conradi	VSD/ PDA
Cockayne	Atherosclerosis
Cutis laxa	Pulmonary hypertension/ PPS
Cystic Fibrosis	Cor Pulmonale
Ellis-Van-Creveld	ASD (usually single atrium)/ Misc.CHD
Friedreich Ataxia	Cardiomyopathy
Glycogenosis [IIa/IIIa/IV]	Cardiomyopathy
Homocystinuria	Coronary and other Vascular thromboses
Jervell-Lange-Nielsen	Prolonged QTc Interval/ Sudden Death [VA]/ Congenital Deafness
Laurence-Moon-Biedl	VSD/ Misc.CHD
Mucolipidosis III	Aortic Valve Disease
Mucopolysaccharidosis [MPS]	
IH [Hurler]	CAD/AR/MR
IS [Scheie]/IV[Morquio]/ VI [Maroteaux-Lamy]	Aortic Valve Disease/ CAD
Osteogenesis imperfecta	Aortic Valve Disease
Progeria	Atherosclerosis
Pseudo-xanthoma elasticum	CAI/ MR/ Hypertension
Riley-Day	Episodic Hypertension/ postural hypotension
Refsum	A-V Conduction Defects
Seckel	VSD/ PDA
Sickle Cell Disease	Cardiomyopathy/ MR
Smith-Lemli-Opitz	VSD/ PDA/ Misc.CHD
Thrombocytopenia/Absent Radius	ASD/ TOF/ Dextrocardia
Thalassemia Major	Cardiomyopathy
Weill-Marchesani	PDA
Werner	Vascular Sclerosis

DOMINANT SYNDROMES:

Apert	VSD/ TOF
Crouzon	PDA/ AC
Ehlers-Danlos	Rupture of large vessels (e.g.carotids)/ Dissecting Ao Aneurysm
Familial Periodic Paralysis	Hypokalemia/PST
Forney	MR
Holt-Oram	ASD/ VSD
Hypertrophic Obstructive Cardiomyopathy [HOCM]	Variable Penetrance of Dynamic Sub-aortic Stenosis
Leopard	PS/ Prolonged PR interval/ abnormal P waves on ECG
Lymphedema[Milroy/Meige]	Lymphedema
Marfan	MVP/ MR/ AR/ Aortic aneurysm with possible dissection or rupture
Myotonic-dystrophy [Steinert]	Cardiomyopathy
Neurofibramotosis	PS/ AC/ Pheochromocytoma
Noonan	PS/ ASD/ HOCM
Osler-Weber-Rendu	Telangiectasias/ Pulmonary A-V Malformations
Osteogenesis Imperfecta	AR
Romano-Ward	Prolonged QTc Interval/ Sudden Death [VA]
Treacher Collins	VSD/ PDA/ ASD
Tuberous sclerosis	Myocardial rhabdomyomata
Von Hippel-Lindau	Hemangiomata/ Pheo-chromocytoma

X-LINKED SYNDROMES [R=Recessive/D=Dominant]:

MPS II [Hunter] R	CAD/Valve Disease
Muscular Dystrophy [Duchenne] R	Cardiomyopathy
Muscular Dystrophy [Dreifuss] R	Cardiomyopathy
Incontinentia pigmenti D	PDA
Goltz D	Occasional Misc.CHD/ Telangiectasia

Key: MR=Mitral Regurgitation/ AR=Aortic Regurgitation/, CAI=Coronary Artery Insufficiency/ CAD=Coronary Artery Disease/ PST=Paroxysmal Supraventricular Tachycardia/ ECD=Endocardial Cushion Defect/ HOCM=Hypertrophic Obstructive Cardiomyopathy/ VA=Ventricular Arrhythmias

Notes

1. Rose VR, Gold RJM, Lindsay G, Allen M: A Possible Increase in the Incidence of Congenital Heart Defects Among the Offspring of Affected Parents. *JACC* 6:376, 1985.

2. Clark EB, Boughman JA, Ferencz C: Familial Risk of Left Heart Defects: A Population Based Epidemiologic Study. AAP Abstract. *Am Heart J* 112:651, 1986.

3. Modified from Fyler DC: Report of the New England Regional Infant Cardiac Program. *Pediatrics* 65:376-471, 1980.

4. Modified from Nora JJ: *Etiological Aspects of Heart Disease.* In Adams FH, Emmanoulides GC (eds): *Heart Disease in Infants, Children, and Adolescents*, 3rd Edition. Baltimore, Williams & Wilkins, 1983, p 2 [With Permission].

5. Katz Z, Lancet M, Skornik J, Chemke J, Mogilner BM, Klinberg, M: Teratogenicity of Progestogens Given During the First Trimester of Pregnancy. *Obstetrics & Gynecology* 65: 775, 1985.

6. Wiseman RA, Dodds-Smith IC: Cardiovascular Birth Defects and Antenatal Exposure to Female Sex Hormones: A Reevaluation of Some Base Data. *Teratology* 30:359, 1984.

7. Modified from Nora JJ: *Etiological Aspects of Heart Disease.* In Adams FH, Emmanoulides GC (eds): *Heart Disease in Infants, Children, and Adolescents*, 3rd Edition. Baltimore, Williams & Wilkins, 1983, p 2 [With Permission].

8. Clark EB, Boughman JA, Ferencz C: Familial Risk of Left Heart Defects: A Population Based Epidemiologic Study. AAP Abstract. *Am Heart J* 112:651, 1986.

9. Ibid.

10. Modified from Nora JJ: *Etiological Aspects of Heart Disease.* In Adams FH, Emmanoulides GC (eds): *Heart Disease in Infants, Children, and Adolescents*, 3rd Edition. Baltimore, Williams & Wilkins, 1983, p 2 [With Permission].

Chapter 2

Cardiac History and Physical Exam

After careful consideration, it appears that the most useful way to present important historical data relating to infants and children with significant cardiac disorders would be to review points in a general pediatric or family practice visit that would "*flag*" a significant reason to seek Pediatric Cardiology consultation. The following is a compilation of complaints or history that could relate to the child's cardio-vascular system. Some are subtle but nevertheless bear mentioning. Possible associations follow the specific historical point for further thought.

[1] Easy Tiring during Feeding: Such a finding is common in infants with congenital cardiac defects or other causes of congestive cardiac failure. During infancy, the greatest activity of the day often involves feeding, and therefore if cardiac reserve is limited, the infant is forced to rest frequently while feeding. The mother and father often comment that "it takes forever for my child to finish a bottle." The group of lesions associated with the most severe forms of congestive cardiac failure include complete atrio-ventricular canal defects/ truncus arteriosus/ very large ventricular septal defects [VSD] or double outlet right ventricle/ severe aortic coarctation especially in association with VSD/ tricuspid atresia with no pulmonary stenosis/ total anomalous pulmonary venous return without obstruction to venous return/ complete transposition with VSD and no pulmonary stenosis.

[2] Poor Weight Gain: With a history of poor feeding it is common to have a parent note that the child is gaining weight poorly, compared with their other children, relatives or neighbors. The same lesions associated with the most serious forms of congestive cardiac failure [CHF] are the same that cause the most severe forms of "cardiac cachexia," which is an extreme of poor weight gain associated with severe chronic CHF, and overt *wasting.*

Increased palmar concavity with loss of fat pads is typical.

[3] Grunting and Rapid Breathing: Pulmonary edema associated with CHF makes it desirable for the infant to attempt to keep terminal airways open in order to preserve as much pulmonary reserve as possible in face of the poorly compliant lungs. The application of positive end expiratory pressure [PEEP] would accomplish this. Innately, the infant with significant CHF grunts almost constantly. This mode of respiration provides some PEEP during breathing. The sound is similar to forced panting, and quite easy to recognize by parents and physicians. Associated with this nearly constant grunting is sustained rapid breathing, often noted again by the parents. In extreme cases, the parents note that "my child's head appears to be bobbing when he breathes." This is a result of the very increased respiratory effort. These symptoms are not to be confused with normal occasional periods of grunting and slightly rapid breathing in many infants, especially during straining with bowel movements.

[4] Easy Diaphoresis [Sweating], Especially during Feeding, and Even in Cool Surroundings: The stressed infant with CHF usually has a marked endogenous catecholamine release, resulting in diaphoresis. It is important to realize that the ability to display diaphoresis develops postnatally, and the young infant less than 2 to 3 months old will not manifest this finding.

[5] Duskiness or Overt Cyanosis: Complex cyanotic congenital heart disease, if not detected in the newborn nursery, usually results in the parents recognition of at least "duskiness" on the lips and buccal mucosa, when questioned carefully. It is important to differentiate this historically from the normal variant acrocyanosis involving distal extremities and the peri-oral regions. This most commonly occurs when the infant is chilled and likely results from immature peripheral vascular tone. Peri-oral cyanosis is a variation of this and does not necessarily imply cyanotic congenital heart disease unless the lips and buccal mucosa are also involved. Rarely cyanosis is caused by methemoglobinemia. In the newborn, persistent fetal circulation, pulmonary disease or pulmonary immaturity are other causes of cyanosis [see separate discussions].

[6] Stridor, Wheezing, or Dysphagia: Although likely associated with other than cardio-vascular etiologies, persistent complaints of *stridor* may be associated with

vascular rings from aortic arch anomalies such as *double aortic arch* and its variants. Persistent and often progressive *wheezing* may result from the rare anomaly of *aberrant left pulmonary artery arising from the right pulmonary artery.* As this artery courses from the right to left, it compresses the trachea at a level associated with wheezing, not stridor as in the vascular ring. The aberrant left pulmonary artery malformation is often named *vascular sling* as opposed to *vascular ring.*

Dysphagia in an older child may result from an unusual form of ordinarily uncomplicated, benign aberrant right subclavian artery, that arises from the descending aorta [assuming a normal left aortic arch]. Truly symptomatic children with this basic vascular anomaly also have *bicarotid truncus* [both carotid arteries arising from a common vessel or in very close proximity]. The additional presence of *an aortic diverticulum* (diverticulum of Kommerell) would further promote esophageal compression with true dysphagia. Unfortunately, American medical literature has not emphasized this interesting cause for true dysphagia, which in the instance of isolated aberrant right subclavian artery would usually be noted as *dysphagia lusoria* [imaginary dysphagia]. One of the most complete monographs about aortic arch anomalies is no longer in print, but does refer to the combination of aberrant right subclavian artery and bicarotid truncus as a cause of true dysphagia (1). Other monographs exist, that also elaborate these anomalies well (2,3).

[7] <u>Apparent Extreme Chest Pain That Awakens a Sleeping Infant</u>: In the rare malformation of aberrant left coronary artery arising from the pulmonary artery, once the high neonatal pulmonary vascular resistance decreases, it is probable that the infant will suffer an antero-lateral myocardial infarction, resulting in the unusual history of unconsolable agitation and apparent pain.

[8] <u>Moderate Chest Pain Usually Unassociated With Exercise:</u> Chest pain in the older child or adolescent is ordinarily not cardiac in origin but rather often represents esophageal spasm or a musculoskeletal condition such as costochondritis or intercostal neuralgia. Increased frequency or severity of esophageal spasm pain is common with iced drinks during the summer, stress, or caffeine as well as theophylline-containing beverages. The pain is usually very severe and mid sternal, without relation to exercise. It passes in several minutes and may be so severe that the patient develops a rapid pulse as well, from

fright. In relation to fright, a relatively newly recognized *panic attack syndrome* has been described in adults as well as in children. This is associated with a *feeling of dread*, *palpitations*, and possible *chest pain*. The patient is usually aware that "my heart is beating very strongly," during such attacks. Also relatively new is Kawasaki Disease which may be associated with coronary artery aneurysms. Rarely these develop thrombotic occlusion with resulting myocardial infarction and therefore myocardial pain. *Cardiomyopathy* and significant *aortic stenosis* may also result in cardiac pain. The rare malformation of *abnormal coronary artery course* [anomalous origin of the left coronary artery from the right sinus of Valsalva or anomalous origin of the right coronary artery from the left sinus of Valsalva] may be associated with anginal chest pain during maximal exercise, and sudden death. Recent evidence suggests that the entity of myocardial bridging or tunneled coronary arteries whereby a portion of a major coronary artery such as the left anterior descending is completely surrounded by myocardium, is likely not associated with sudden death or angina [see discussion of sudden cardiac death]. Non-specific chest pain attributed to mitral valve prolapse is relatively common in adult patients but somewhat unusual in children. This pain is not anginal in nature and responds to propranolol therapy.

In summary, chest pain is most often not cardiac in origin, but rare cardiac etiologies to chest pain do exist in children. Careful attention as to whether the chest pain is associated with exercise, its maximal location, quality, distribution, and duration as well as methods of relief, is critical to decide whether its origin is likely cardiac or not. For example, aspirin has been found by experience to be very helpful for intercostal neuralgia and costochondritis. If used to try to control pain from these causes, one must observe the usual pediatric precautions about aspirin and its relation to Reye's Syndrome. Although a common cause for non-specific chest pain in the adult, mitral valve prolapse *ordinarily does not cause* frequent chest pain in children, even though it is extremely common.

[9] <u>Palpitations, Dizziness, or Syncope</u>: Complaints of palpitations in children usually relate to benign cardiac dysrhythmias; nevertheless every effort must be made to document the exact dysrhythmia if possible. There are now intermittent transtelephonic ECG recording units that are most helpful in documenting brief episodes of dysrhythmias in children. Dizziness in not commonly associated with

palpitations in children and if present, suggests a more significant cardiac dysrhythmia. Syncope may be vaso-vagal in origin in children, but one must keep in mind the ominous ventricular dysrhythmias potentially associated with *Prolonged QT Interval Syndrome*. Although baseline ECG may have a normal QTc interval, one may be able to demonstrate a prolonged QT interval in such patients during vagal maneuvers or during exercise. If syncope is secondary to ventricular dysrhythmias associated with prolonged QTc interval, therapy with agents such as phenytoin or propranolol must be attempted. Dysrhythmias associated with *hypertrophic obstructive cardiomyopathy* are also usually serious, and one should rule this out in most children with cardiac dysrhythmias.

Rarely syncope relates to sudden complete A-V block in children, although patients with corrected transposition [L-loop, ventricular inversion] may develop increasing degrees of A-V block. Children who have had surgical correction of complex cardiac malformation are also at risk of syncope and sudden death. Fortunately this is not common, but cannot be dismissed.

[10] Hyperdynamic Cardiac Impulse: Although ordinarily a physical finding on exam, it is not uncommon for alert parents or grandparents to convey that "my child's heart seems as though it's coming out of the chest, it beats so vigorously." This finding is usually noted upon placing the child over the shoulder after feeding, and corresponds to a hyperdynamic precordial impulse secondary to a significant congenital malformation of the heart. Such a finding is associated with increased left to right shunt flow. The prominent precordial impulses associated with cyanotic forms of CHD such as VSD with severe pulmonary stenosis are more sustained or thrusting in quality, not truly hyperdynamic. The finding of a hyperdynamic precordial impulse is often ignored and yet may be the only clue that a significant cardiac defect exists.

[11] Exercise Intolerance in the Older Child: Poor exercise ability is usually not cardiac in origin in older children, unless they have evidence for overt CHF or cardiomyopathy. Rarely, the child with a large Atrial Septal Defect will complain of exercise intolerance, but this complaint is much more typical for the adult with such a defect.

[12] Frequent Upper Respiratory Infections [URI] and Pneumonias: Children with increased pulmonary blood flow from a congenital heart defect often have decreased lung

compliance. There is an association of increased pulmonary blood flow and frequent uri and possible pneumonias. Such an association is not present in patients with decreased pulmonary blood flow, as in tetralogy of Fallot. These patients are at some slight risk, however, of pulmonary thrombosis.

[13] Swollen, Peeling Fingers with Angular Stomatitis, Significant Temperature Elevation, Fretfulness, Swollen Glands and Thrombocytosis: These historical findings are consistent with Kawasaki Disease which may be associated with coronary artery aneurysms per [8] above, under chest pain.

[14] Dizziness Upon Vigorous Exercise Involving the Upper Extremities: Rarely, a *subclavian steal syndrome* secondary to stenotic origin of the subclavian artery from an aortic arch anomaly, results in this unusual form of dizziness associated with vigorous upper extremity activity.

[15] Arthritis, Arthralgia, Fever, Stomach Pain, Clumsiness (Sydenham Chorea): Although very rare now, *Acute Rheumatic Fever* (ARF) often presents with one or more of the above historical complaints. The diagnosis should still be considered if lab data further suggest recent Group A, beta hemolytic streptococcal pharyngitis. The finding of Sydenham Chorea itself, allows one to make a diagnosis of ARF in a child, and is such a late manifestation that there is seldom evidence for streptococcal pharyngitis at the time of presentation (see discussion of ARF).

[16] Upper Airway Obstruction (Snoring, Marked Difficulty Breathing on an Upper Airway Basis): This entity may become serious enough to result in overt Cor Pulmonale. In early stages, ECG abnormalities may be present such as *right atrial abnormality, prominent anterior and/or rightward forces, borderline right axis deviation.*

[17] Congenital nerve deafness [Jervell-Lange-Nielsen]: There is an association between congenital deafness and prolonged QT interval Syndrome with possible syncope and sudden death. See further discussion under [9] above.

[18] High dietary salt intake: Occasionally a child with such a history presents with a hyperdynamic circulation manifesting prominent precordial impulses, prominent peripheral pulses, and suggestive diastolic overload on the ECG. Careful determination of blood pressures in such

children is also important, especially if there is a family history of hypertension.

[19] Important Perinatal History: Infants of diabetic mothers are at higher than usual risk of congenital heart disease and often develop transient, but significant cardiomyopathy. They also have a tendency to develop hypoglycemia and hypocalcemia both of which tend to compromise newborn myocardial function significantly.

Prematurity is associated with a high incidence of PDA, often associated with physiological peripheral pulmonary stenosis. *Neonatal asphyxia* especially on the basis of meconium aspiration with hypoglycemia or hypocalcemia or polycythemia often relates to the development of *persistent fetal circulation* and associated cyanosis. Maternal exposure to agents listed in Table 1.2 should alert the house staff that there is a greater chance that the newborn may have a significant cardiac malformation. Maternal lupus erythematosis has an association with complete heart block in the infant. This is often noted pre-natally.

[20] Important Family Cardiovascular History: This includes any history of *initial myocardial infarction in men specifically less than 50 years of age or in women less than 60 years of age*. If this history is positive, the parent in whose family this occurred, should be screened with a 12 - 16 hour fasting serum cholesterol and triglyceride level. If positive or if the family member is the mother or father, the child should have similar screening. Statistically 30% of families with such histories will have familial hyperlipoproteinemia.

First degree family members with congenital cardiac defects should be recorded. Positive family histories of hypertension, sudden death, obesity, cardiac dysrhythmias, and cardiomyopathy are all relevant.

Just as with "*flags*" in the pediatric history, there are "*flags*" in a careful pediatric exam that should indicate a significant or subtle problem with the cardiovascular system. Below is a list of important points relating to a thorough pediatric C-V exam.

[1] General Appearance and Inspection Including Evidence for a Genetic Disorder: Basically one first needs to know whether the child is comfortable at rest and whether there are findings consistent with a known genetic disorder such

as *Down Syndrome*. Based upon the 50% occurrence of congenital cardiac malformations in such children, it is common for a pediatrician or family practitioner to seek cardiology consultation even prior to discharge from the nursery. Echocardiography definitively rules out a large VSD or complete atrio-ventricular canal defect which is common in this group of children. Physical exam could be quite benign in the neonatal period because the high neonatal pulmonary vascular resistance prevents a large left to right shunt and increase in pulmonary blood flow. Even if murmurs do not exist, the infant with Down Syndrome could have a large, significant cardiac defect. Other important genetic disorders include *Marfan Syndrome*, *Noonan Syndrome*, and any others that are associated with an increased risk of cardiac disorders (see Table 1.4). The infant of a diabetic mother also has an increased incidence of congenital cardiac malformations as well as transient cardiomyopathy.

- Distress associated with cardiac failure is ordinarily respiratory in nature with overt *grunting*, *tachypnea*, *intercostal and subcostal retractions*, *flaring of the ala nasae*. *Diaphoresis* develops with slight crying or agitation. If chronic, there is associated evidence of failure to thrive with possible cachexia. Many cardiologists have noted that infants with *total anomalous pulmonary venous return* appear very *tall* and underweight. Height is preserved whereas the increased metabolic demands result in poor weight gain. In more severe forms of CHF, height is also affected. Infants with cardiac failure are ordinarily very fretful, difficult to console and anxious. Cyanosis may or may not be present, depending upon the duration and severity of CHF. If present, cyanosis is usually mild and associated with a *dusky* appearance, because of poor cardiac output. It is interesting that the severe forms of cyanotic congenital heart disease are those that are rarely associated with congestive failure, with the exception of complete transposition of the great vessels with VSD. Infants with severe pulmonary stenosis and VSD (tetralogy of Fallot), may be markedly cyanotic, but do not develop CHF.

If chronic, cardiac volume overload often results in left precordial prominence (assuming that dextrocardia is not present). This finding is often noted by the family and may be best assessed with the child in a reclining position.

If truly present, *central cyanosis* should be assessed by observing the tongue, lips and buccal mucosa. Even in the black infant, one should be able to recognize cyanosis in these regions. One should differentiate *central cyanosis* from the normal variant *acrocyanosis* presenting with significant peripheral cyanosis on the hands and feet and possibly in the peri-oral region. This form of cyanosis is common if the infant is cold and is not associated with central cyanosis. The etiology is probably peripheral vasomotor immaturity. Rarely it takes many months to one year for such peripheral cyanosis to disappear. Infants with *hypoplastic left heart syndromes* are usually not overtly cyanotic, but rather *gray in appearance*, because of markedly reduced systemic cardiac output.

Clubbing of the extremities develops in cyanotic children over several years, and unfortunately does not disappear after corrective surgery. This finding in the adult may be associated with severe pulmonary dysfunction in lieu of cyanotic heart disease. It may also be benign and familial.

One should carefully note thoracic skeletal configuration. Patients with pectus excavatum configuration, straight back syndrome, narrow thoracic A-P diameter, and thoracic scoliosis all have a higher than usual incidence of mitral valve prolapse. In such patients, careful attention to the presence of apical systolic clicks is important. Depending upon the source, as many as *12-16% of women and 8% of men have this usually benign condition.*

A *large tongue* in an infant with a *short PR interval on the ECG* may be a clue to *glycogen storage disease* with its associated cardiomyopathy.

Skin manifestations of neurofibromatosis or of Leopard syndrome may be a clue to underlying cardiac pathology.

Pedal edema or presacral edema is not present in infants with CHF, but rather, subtle edema of the dorsa of the hands and feet may be present in these children.

[2] Vital Signs: Normal heart and respiratory rates are good evidence against cardiac compromise. Cardiac rhythm should be noted during auscultation and irregularities mentioned. A normal sinus arrhythmia is most common, whereby there is an increase in rate during inspiration with a decrease in rate at the beginning of expiration. Blood pressures should be obtained in upper and lower extremities. If the child is very small, flush blood pressures are acceptable. Do not forget that systolic

pressure in the legs is usually 10-15 mm. Hg. higher than in the arms, because of pulse wave reflection along the aorta in children. This phenomenon does not exist in adults.

[3] Palpation: Simple palpation remains a very useful and important part of the complete pediatric cardiac exam. *Pulses in all four extremities should be carefully palpated to assess quality and symmetry*. Patients with PDA ordinarily have full-volume bounding pulses with easy to palpate dorsalis pedis and posterior tibial pulses. Patients with VSD often have prominent peripheral pulses on the basis of rapid-upstroke, not volume. Occasionally one may appreciate the classical *pulsus bisferens* [bimodal pulse] associated with severe forms of hypertrophic obstructive cardiomyopathy. Peripheral pulses are usually decreased in children with congestive heart failure. Older literature states that subtly decreased pulses exist in children with ASD, but the author has not noted this finding in his clinical practice. Decreased pulses may be the only clue to the existence of hypoplastic left heart syndrome in the otherwise stable neonate, although these infants usually present with a gray color from very diminished cardiac output.

Decreased or absent femoral pulses exist in infants and children with aortic coarctation. One must be very alert and realize that in the immediate newborn period, aortic coarctation may not manifest with decreased femoral pulses because the PDA is still opened [see discussion about aortic coarctation]. In the older child with long-standing aortic coarctation, collateral flow around the obstruction may result in relatively easily palpable femoral pulses. However, astute recognition of a delay in the femoral pulses is possible if one palpates the right radial and right femoral pulses simultaneously. This finding of *radial-femoral pulse lag* represents the longer transit time of the central aortic pulse through the long, tortuous collateral vessels. At this point in the natural history of aortic coarctation, one also might palpate interscapular pulsations secondary to collateral vessel flow.

Unilateral decrease in upper extremity pulses is quite unusual but could be associated with stenotic origin of a subclavian artery associated with an aortic arch anomaly. The possibility of such a finding makes its imperative to palpate all four extremity pulses, without exception. It is unfortunate that it remains fairly common for a patient to present in late childhood with significant systemic hypertension secondary to previously undetected aortic coarctation.

While assessing peripheral pulses it is reasonable to indirectly assess peripheral perfusion by pressing firmly in an area of an extremity and observing the rapidity of refill. Experience will allow accurate determination of whether peripheral perfusion is significantly decreased, if this becomes a routine, even in normal exams. Decreased perfusion is usually present in the child with congestive cardiac failure.

Cardiac evaluation involves abdominal palpation, usually limited to determination of hepatomegaly and the nature of the hepatic margin. The liver edge is ordinarily palpated 1-2 cm. below the right costal margin in the infant and young child and has an easily defined sharp edge. Once again experience will allow the house officer to accurately assess a normal liver edge. Subtly, with low grade chronic CHF, the liver may not be overtly enlarged, yet upon careful palpation one might recognize a dull, rounded liver margin, consistent with chronic, low grade CHF. Do not assume that the liver will be present beneath the right costal margin. With situs inversus and with the complex asplenia/ polysplenia syndromes, the liver may be in the left sub-costal region or in a horizontal mid sub-costal position. Unusually, splenic enlargement relates to the C-V system. Myocarditis associated with mononucleosis and cardiac sequelae to sickle cell disease are two examples.

<u>Cardiac and Precordial Palpation:</u> One should perform precordial palpation with the patient in a reclining position approaching the thorax from the right side, and using the right hand to ensure consistent examinations. Using the finger tips, it is usually possible to appreciate the apical impulse. In the immediate newborn period this may be difficult. The apical impulse is usually palpated at or just medial to the mid-left clavicular line in the fourth intercostal space in the young infant. The intercostal space associated with the apical impulse increases to the fifth and sixth interspace as the child grows older. If the apical impulse is displaced leftward [laterally], then one has evidence for cardiomegaly. In left to right shunt lesions resulting in LV volume overload such as VSD/ PDA/ or complete A-V Canal, the apical impulse is *hyperdynamic*. In left to right shunt lesions resulting in RV volume overload such as ASD, the RV impulse is very hyperdynamic at the lower left and mid sternal border. The RV impulse is best palpated with the mid-palmar region

placed at the mid to lower left sternal border. Lesions resulting in pressure overload of either ventricle, result in a prominent, thrusting impulse in the respective ventricular regions, as opposed to the very dynamic impulse described above. These findings are very important, not only as a quick means to assess cardiomegaly, but as an indication that something may be wrong with the heart. *It is quite unlikely that a very serious cardiac defect exists if one is able to palpate a quiet cardiac impulse with no lateral displacement of the apical impulse.* Furthermore, the finding of a prominent RV impulse may be the only clue to the existence of an ASD in an otherwise unremarkable cardiac exam. As noted in history, above, it is possible for the family to note precordial hyperactivity in infants with serious congenital cardiac defects when the infants are placed over the shoulder after feeding. *Every normal pediatric exam should include the simple precordial palpation.* Note the use of the term apical impulse in lieu of PMI [point of maximal impulse]. Most pediatric cardiologists prefer this term to describe palpation of the most lateral ventricle because in many children with congenital cardiac defects, the true maximal impulse is the RV heave at the lower left sternal border. Finally, do not forget to palpate the right precordium if a cardiac impulse is not readily palpable on the left. Children may have dextrocardia. Auscultation of the heart over the right hemi-thorax would also be more distinct in these instances.

After establishing the quality of cardiac impulses one must palpate the precordial region for evidence of thrills, which are no more than a reflection of a loud murmur. Typically thrills associated with VSD are maximal at the lower left sternal border. Those associated with pulmonary stenosis are located over the pulmonary area at the upper left sternal border, whereas aortic stenosis often results in a systolic thrill over the aortic area at the upper right sternal border. Older literature suggests that peak systolic pressure differences less than 25 mm. Hg are usually not associated with systolic thrills in cases of pulmonary or aortic valvar stenosis. The author has appreciated rare systolic thrills in patients with aortic stenosis associated with a systolic pressure difference of 15 mm. Hg during cardiac cath. Note that this entity would be assessed non-invasively, now, by Doppler study, and cath would be limited only to those children with stenosis in the range that could require surgery or interventional cath. *One should always include the supra-sternal notch region in methodical palpation.* Lesions that might result in a systolic thrill in this particular region include:

aortic stenosis/ pulmonary stenosis/ aortic coarctation/ PDA. PDA may also result in a systolic thrill in the left infra-clavicular area. In addition to systolic thrills, in unusual instances where extreme pulmonary hypertension exists, one would be able to actually palpate the pulmonary component of the second heart at the upper left sternal border. A hyperdynamic pulmonary artery may also be palpated in this region, if one palpates carefully.

Percussion: Percussion of the left border of cardiac dullness truly has no place in pediatric cardiology because of the very small thorax in the infant and child. This maneuver was commonly performed by the careful practitioner trying to assess whether cardiomegaly existed in the older patient. In such a case, one would find lateral displacement of the left cardiac border. If one further noted that in spite of the displacement of the left cardiac border to percussion, the apical impulse was in a normal position by palpation, one might conclude that the patient had a moderate pericardial effusion accounting for this discrepancy. All this clinical information was possible in days before echocardiography!

[4] Auscultation of the Lungs: The lungs are usually quite clear in most children with a cardiac malformation unless it is associated with significant congestive heart failure. In this case, one may appreciate a bronchial pattern of breathing rather than broncho-vesicular (duration of inspiratory phase = to that of expiratory phase, in lieu of greater duration of inspiratory phase, as is normal). This finding is very subtle. Overt wheezing is not common in children with CHF, but is occasionally present. Stridor or wheezing may suggest the presence of a vascular ring or vascular sling (see under history). Basal rales are also uncommon in infants and children with CHF, but may be present in the older child in heart failure. Pleural friction rubs are possible as a part of the post-pericardiotomy syndrome and should be assessed carefully.

[5] Auscultation of the Heart: The art of cardiac auscultation appears to be less emphasized with the advent of sophisticated non-invasive evaluation by echocardiography and by cardiac doppler. However, if the practicing pediatrician or family practitioner fails to maintain cardiac auscultatory skills, failure to recognize a potentially fatal cardiac malformation becomes possible. The simplest example would be failure to appreciate the single quality of the second heart sound in patients with hypoplastic left heart syndrome, in patients with complete

transposition, or in patients with severe pulmonary stenosis and VSD. *The primary care physician should make every effort to determine that the second heart sound in a given child or infant is at least physiologically split and further has a normal pulmonary component for age.* Although the second heart sound often appears single in the immediate newborn period, by the time of usual discharge from the newborn nursery at two to three days, the second heart sound is then usually split allowing appreciation of both the aortic and pulmonary components.

The first heart sound [S1]: Even with the most complex congenital cardiac malformations, the first heart sound is most often normal. However, in children with common A-V canal defects, the first heart sound is often increased because of the abnormal structure of the mitral and tricuspid valves. With VSD, the systolic murmur may be so long as to even render the first heart sound indistinct. PR interval on the ECG directly relates to the intensity of the first heart sound in most instances where no other cardiac pathology exists. *Prolonged PR interval* [first degree A-V block] is associated with a *decreased intensity* of the first heart sound, presumably because this timing allows the A-V valves to float back to a more closed position before the period of iso-volumic ventricular contraction, and hence the sound associated with their closing [S1] is less intense. Using similar reasoning, a *short PR interval* is associated with an *increased intensity* of the first heart sound because the A-V valves are at their relative maximal separation at the time of iso-volumic contraction and therefore create a louder S1 upon closing. Hence, the very clever physician might suspect a pre-excitation syndrome such as Wolf-Parkinson-White or Lown-Ganong-Levine syndromes, upon appreciating an increased S1. This finding should be carefully assessed in the child with a history of palpitation, because pre-excitation syndromes are one cause of cardiac dysrhythmias in children.

Cardiomyopathy in young children often presents with distant "pitter-patter" heart sounds because of the marked decrease in myocardial contractility. Occasionally, marked pericardial effusion presents with distant or muffled heart sounds as well. It is unfortunately not uncommon for the physician to ignore these findings because of their rarity.

The second heart sound [S2]: *Correct auscultation of the second heart sound is probably the most difficult responsibility of the primary care physician relative to an accurate cardiac exam*. Yet with proper orientation, each physician should be able to at least determine whether two components of the second heart sound exist. The appreciation of physiological splitting of the second heart sound at least conveys the fact that the child has an aortic valve and a pulmonic valve. Absence or severe stenosis of a semi-lunar valve results in absence of the component of the second heart sound associated with that valve. In children with hypoplastic left heart syndrome and aortic atresia, the second heart sound must be single, because there is no functioning aortic valve. Similarly, in children with severe tetralogy of Fallot, the pulmonary stenosis is so severe that the pulmonary component of the second heart sound becomes inaudible. In infants with truncus arteriosus, there is only one semi-lunar valve and ordinarily a loud single second heart sound, as well. Occasionally in this group of patients, the truncal valve is so complex (possibly associated with four or five leaflets), that one could have the impression that the second heart sound is truly split. A precordial hyperdynamic impulse, mild cyanosis, bounding pulses, and a possible systolic click because of truncal dilatation might still indicate to the examining physician that something is wrong with the heart, even if the second heart sound appeared slightly split. In infants with *complete transposition of the great vessels*, although two semilunar valves exist, the aortic valve is very anterior and to the right of the pulmonary valve. Because of the more distant location of the pulmonary valve and the more proximal location of the aortic valve in these infants, *the classical auscultatory finding becomes a loud, single second heart sound* representing the aortic component. Using the above principles, one could basically determine whether a given child had a potentially serious cardiac problem. Children with ASD present with widely split second heart sounds that do not vary significantly with respiration [widely split, fixed second heart sound]. This finding and an RV heave at the lower left sternal border may be the clue that an ASD exists. *Assessment of the second heart sound should be done with the child in a sitting position in the older child, because it is common for the second heart sound to appear prominently split during reclining* because of the change in venous return in this position. Children with total anomalous pulmonary venous return also have widely split and fixed second heart sounds if there is no obstruction to pulmonary venous return. Similarly, partial anomalous venous return with intact atrial septum may be associated with widely split second heart sounds. Complete right bundle branch block also relates to a widely split S2. However, in this case one may appreciate slight physiological movement.

Not only is it possible to appreciate splitting of the second heart sound, but one can also assess the intensity of the two components. *In comparing the aortic component with the pulmonary component of the second heart sound one should listen solely in the pulmonary area for consistency of examination.* In this region, the louder aortic component [A2] may be heard and compared with the pulmonary component [P2]. In the neonate, this high pulmonary vascular resistance results in pulmonary hypertension and therefore the pulmonary component of S2 is accordingly increased. It is important to realize that dependent left to right shunts such as VSD/ PDA or even common A-V Canal may not manifest physiologically or on exam until the high neonatal vascular resistance decreases by approximately four to eight weeks of age. Any cause for increased pulmonary artery pressures results in an increased intensity to the second heart sound. For example in a child with otherwise uncomplicated VSD, if P2 is not increased, it is evidence that the VSD is restrictive to pressure and therefore not very large. In cases where a large VSD is balanced by moderate to severe pulmonary stenosis, P2 would again not be increased, but rather decreased or absent. Moderate stenotic lesions of the pulmonary valve result in a decreased P2, associated with more wide splitting of S2 because of the increased time of RV ejection secondary to obstruction. With aortic stenosis, one may appreciate a more narrowly split second heart sound because of the increased LV ejection period. In unusually severe instances of aortic stenosis, the second heart sound may even appear paradoxically split [during inspiration there is less splitting of the second heart sound rather than increased splitting as is normal]. The usual explanation of why the second heart sound splits physiologically involves the increased time necessary for the RV to eject its increased volume during inspiration, when the intrathoracic pressure becomes more negative and promotes increased systemic venous return. At the same time, inspiration is associated with slightly retarded pulmonary venous emptying and therefore the LV has slightly less volume to deal with, decreasing LV ejection time. Therefore during inspiration, the pulmonary component of the second heart sound occurs later and the aortic component occurs earlier, resulting in a more widely split S2. With increasing degrees of pulmonary hypertension, the second heart sound becomes more narrowly split, likely because the RV faces similar afterload compared with the LV, when pulmonary artery pressures and resistance increase. Therefore one could appreciate more narrowly split second heart sounds with both aortic stenosis and with pulmonary hypertension such as with large VSD. In the latter situation, however, the intensity of the second heart sound would also be increased. In the infant with left sided obstructive lesions such as severe aortic stenosis or aortic coarctation, pulmonary vascular resistance and pressures also increase significantly and therefore in this age range, such lesions are associated with increased pulmonary components of the second heart sound and more narrow splitting.

In summary, careful attention to the splitting of the second heart sound and to the intensity of the individual components of that sound is critical in the accurate assessment of the pediatric cardiovascular exam. Increased skills in this area might relate to an ability to detect critical forms of congenital heart disease that otherwise could be missed.

The Third Heart Sound [S3]: It is quite common to appreciate the presence of a normal third heart sound in children. However, if a third heart sound newly appears in a child that previously did not have this finding, one must be suspicious for possible early CHF as the cause of this finding. In overt CHF, the appreciation of a third heart sound is common and its disappearance under these circumstances indirectly suggests some control of the CHF after starting therapy. Third heart sounds are also common in children with diastolic overload such as exists with ASD. The author has also noticed this finding in children with a marked intake of exogenous salt in their diet [e.g., with cravings for pickles, olives, or potato chips]. Associated with this increased sodium intake are hyperdynamic precordial impulse, full volume pulses, and ECG suggestive of diastolic overload.

Fourth Heart Sound [S4]: The presence of a fourth heart sound, just before the appearance of S1, is *not* a normal finding in children and indicates that the atria are having difficulty filling the ventricles. Causes include cardiomyopathy with decreased ventricular compliance, severe semi-lunar valve stenosis, severe aortic coarctation, endocardial fibroelastosis.

Systolic Clicks: One of the most interesting sounds on cardiac auscultation is the systolic click. Early or ejection systolic clicks were originally described in patients with mild to moderate aortic or pulmonary valve stenosis. With aortic stenosis the click is usually constant and in the region of the aortic valve, whereas the click is usually intermittent and in the region of the pulmonary valve with pulmonary stenosis. With more severe forms of semi-lunar valve stenosis, the valve is so immobile that it cannot generate a click. Bicuspid aortic valve is also associated with a distinct systolic ejection click over the aortic area or along an axis between the apex and aortic region [LV ejection pathway]. Interestingly, 6% of the population has uncomplicated bicuspid aortic valve, based upon necropsy studies.

Other causes of systolic clicks include great vessel dilatation. In patients with tetralogy of Fallot, the pulmonary valve is usually too stenotic to generate a click; however, the aorta is quite dilated because it accepts the usual systemic output in addition to the right to left shunt. In such children one almost always appreciates a systolic click at the mid left sternal border, as a result of aortic dilatation. This finding is also common with truncus arteriosus, as noted above. In the instance of pulmonary hypertension, the dilated pulmonary artery may be associated with a click in the pulmonary region. Transient ventricular septal aneurysm formation upon spontaneous VSD closure often results in a transient systolic ejection click at the mid left sternal border.

The most common etiology for systolic clicks is mitral valve prolapse. With this entity the systolic click is often still early and its maximal location is between the apex and lower left sternal border or at the apex. It is usually loudest with the patient sitting. In the classical form the click is non-ejection and heard in mid systole. Multiple clicks are often present in the classical form of mitral valve prolapse, but this is less common in children. It is now recognized that tricuspid valve prolapse is another etiology for systolic clicks and may co-exist with mitral valve prolapse. The nature of the systolic clicks from tricuspid or mitral valve prolapse appear similar, except for a slightly more medial location of tricuspid prolapse clicks. At least 5% of patients from the general population have mitral valve prolapse and some echo studies suggest an incidence in females as high as 12-16% with an incidence in males of 8%. *Importantly, SBE prophylaxis is indicated for all of the above etiologies for systolic clicks.* In the rarely reported instance of idiopathic dilatation of the main pulmonary artery associated with a systolic click, SBE prophylaxis is likely not necessary.

The Cardiac Murmurs: Placing this physical finding last in the discussion of cardiac auscultation puts it in its proper perspective, because it is often not a cardiac murmur that is the important finding on cardiac exam, but rather all of the more subtle findings as discussed above. Too often a house officer relates a cardiac exam by proudly describing the cardiac murmur and not even noting whether the precordial impulses were normal.

Innocent Vibratory Systolic Ejection Murmur or Still's Murmur: The most common murmur during childhood is the innocent medium to high pitched vibratory Still's murmur. This murmur is particularly evanescent, sometimes present and other times not. It can appear at any age, but is slightly uncommon during infancy. Increased cardiac output associated with fever, anxiety, infection, or exercise, increases the intensity of the murmur which is usually between a Grade 2-3/6 intensity. Its location is very varied, along the left sternal border, at the apex, and possibly even over the aortic area. If loud, it is obviously heard over large areas of the precordium. Its duration is usually short, and its quality is very distinct and somewhat like a *cooing dove*. Once heard, this murmur should be easily identifiable by any well trained physician. *With no other overtones besides vibratory qualities, the examining physician can be assured that the murmur is innocent.* With slightly harsh overtones, one must consider a covert obstructive cardiomyopathy and further evaluation is necessary. Older literature describes an innocent pulmonary ejection murmur which is also short, but maximal in the pulmonary area. It is not harsh, but rather soft or blowing in quality. In the author's experience, with the correct stethoscope one is usually able to appreciate a vibratory quality to this basal innocent systolic ejection murmur, especially with the bell of the stethoscope. This finding of a vibratory quality puts the innocent pulmonary ejection murmur in the category of Still's murmur as well. Slightly more harsh qualities to an ejection murmur in the pulmonary area suggest true pulmonary valve stenosis or atrial septal defect. With pulmonary stenosis there is an associated systolic ejection click and with atrial septal defect the second heart sound is widely split and fixed during respiration.

A harsh, systolic ejection murmur in the aortic region with superior radiation toward the neck is consistent with aortic stenosis.

Extremely common in children is a continuous roaring, *venous hum* in either or both infraclavicular areas with the child sitting only. This murmur which occupies most of systole and spills considerably into diastole, has a distinct quality and again once recognized should be a repeatable assessment. This murmur changes quality with external jugular compression [may disappear] and with change in neck position. Importantly it disappears upon assuming a reclining position. This differs from the continuous, "rocky," PDA murmur located in the left infraclavicular area with possible radiation to the left sternal border, which does not disappear upon reclining or with change in neck position and is often present in the back as well. The term continuous murmur is confusing to the novice, and implies only that the murmur spills past the S2 to enter the diastolic phase, not that the murmur continues throughout systole and diastole. *Continuous murmurs with longer diastolic components are possible from coronary arterio-venous malformations and from the unusual aberrant origin of the left coronary artery from the pulmonary artery.* The longer diastolic component with these forms of continuous murmurs relates to maximal coronary arterial flow during diastole. The murmurs from ventricular septal defect associated with aortic insufficiency were originally described as being continuous in quality, but in reality there is a gap between the VSD quality murmur and the early decrescendo, diastolic blowing murmur of aortic insufficiency. *One must not omit auscultation of the head in an infant with severe unexplained cardiac failure.* The etiology could be cerebral arterio-venous malformation [vein of Galen aneurysm], associated with a continuous murmur upon auscultation over the head [usually maximal in the temporal regions].

An innocent murmur noted especially in the neonate is the slightly harsh Grade 2-3/6 minimally long systolic ejection murmur maximal over the pulmonary area with distinct lateral radiation to both axillae [left often more than right]. This *murmur of physiological peripheral pulmonary stenosis* radiates to the back as well. It relates to the relatively acute angles of origin of the right and left pulmonary arteries from the main pulmonary artery during this age and usually resolves by 18 months to 2 years of age when the pulmonary arterial origins are less acute.

Murmurs associated with very small PDA may be quite short. They are slightly harsh, distinct and ejection in quality with maximal location in the left infraclavicular area. Normal splitting of the second heart sound and normal intensity of the pulmonary component of S2 support the feeling that the PDA is small, if present.

The classical VSD quality murmur is usually a raspy, nearly holosystolic murmur, and maximal at the lower left sternal border with radiation to the right. If the murmur is also present in the left infraclavicular area, the VSD may be present in a supracristal area. What most texts fail to mention is the spectrum of cardiac murmurs associated with large and small VSD. The very large VSD [nearly common ventricle] may have no specific associated systolic murmur. Similarly, a complete A-V canal defect may have such a large VSD that no specific systolic murmur is present. With smaller VSD, the murmur becomes shorter and more ejection in quality until just prior to spontaneous closure, it assumes a very "squirty" quality. *The "squirty" quality to a short systolic ejection murmur maximal at the LLSB should enable the diagnosis of small, closing VSD.* In the case of large VSD with severe infundibular PS, the ejection murmur is usually longer, and more harsh, although occasionally there is a slight "squirty" quality. Once again, absence of an RV heave, and appreciation of a normal S2/P2, support a benign small VSD etiology to a "squirty" murmur, rather than VSD with PS.

The systolic murmur associated with tetralogy of Fallot is the pulmonary stenosis murmur at the mid to upper left sternal border. Serial decreases in the intensity of the basal systolic murmur associated with tetralogy suggest increasing severity of pulmonary stenosis.

Aortic coarctation ordinarily allows detection of a non-specific relatively short systolic ejection murmur over the left posterior hemi-thorax, if some flow is present across the region of narrowing. In about 60% of children with aortic coarctation, a bicuspid aortic valve is present, accounting for an aortic systolic click.

Diastolic murmurs are less common in children and include the murmurs of aortic or pulmonary insufficiency which manifest as early, decrescendo, echoing, blowing diastolic murmurs over the aortic or pulmonary regions. In the case of aortic insufficiency, the diastolic murmur may be heard anywhere along the LV ejection pathway, between the aortic area and the apex. Diastolic rumbles represent excessive flow across one of the A-V valves and are very low pitched, occupying mid diastole and best heard with the bell of the stethoscope. In the case of ASD where the flow increases across the tricuspid valve, the diastolic rumble is maximal at the LLSB, whereas it is maximal at the apex with large VSD where the increased flow is across the mitral valve, from the increased pulmonary blood flow with intact atrial septum. Physiologically, we believe that a diastolic rumble with VSD indicates a greater than 2:1 pulmonary to systemic flow ratio. With ASD, pulmonary to systemic flow ratios usually exceed 2:1 [see physiology section].

An interesting, unusual murmur is the *systolic honk* or *whoop*, which represents mild mitral insufficiency associated with mitral valve prolapse. It is extremely distinct in quality and does sound something likely a honking goose. This rare murmur may be so loud as to be heard by other people in a quiet room, and is usually maximal with the patient sitting.

There are further discussions of murmurs under the various, specific congenital or acquired cardiac malformations, but the above listings cover the major points. Tables 2.1 and 2.2 below, present a synopsis of important cardiac historical and physical exam correlates.

Notes

1. Klinkhamer AC: *Esophagography in Anomalies of the Aortic Arch System*. Baltimore, The Williams & Wilkins Company, 1969.

2. Shuford WH, Sybers RG: *The Aortic Arch and Its Malformations.* Springfield, Charles C Thomas, 1974.

3. Stewart, JR, Kincaid OW, Edwards JE: *An Atlas of Vascular Rings and Related Malformations of the Aortic Arch System*. Springfield, Charles C Thomas, 1964.

Table 2.1: Important Historical Cardiac Correlations

History or Observation	Correlation
IMPORTANT PATIENT HISTORY	
Easy tiring during feeding, poor weight gain, grunting and rapid breathing, easy diaphoresis [sweating], especially during feeding, even in cool surroundings	Classical history suggesting CHF in an infant
Duskiness or overt cyanosis	Probable cyanotic congenital heart defect; consider possible pulmonary disease or persistent fetal circulation in the neonate
Stridor or dysphagia	Consider vascular ring or unusual form of aberrant right subclavian artery
Wheezing	Consider vascular sling [aberrant left pulmonary artery arising from right pulmonary artery]
Apparent, extreme chest pain that awakens a sleeping infant	Possible aberrant left coronary artery arising from the pulmonary artery; pain represents true myocardial infarction
Moderate chest pain usually unassociated with exercise	Consider esophageal spasm, costochondritis, intercostal neuralgia, or cardiomyopathy
Hyperdynamic cardiac impulse	Consider significant left to right shunt as occurs with ventricular or atrial septal defects

Table 2.1: (Continued)

History or Observation	Correlation
Frequent upper respiratory infections [URI] and/or pneumonias	Consider cardiac lesion that causes a high pulmonary blood flow such as ventricular or atrial septal defect
Swollen, peeling fingers with angular stomatitis, significant fever, fretfulness, swollen glands [and thrombocytosis]	Classical findings of Kawasaki Disease
Dizziness upon vigorous exercise of the upper extremities only	Consider subclavian steal syndrome
Arthritis, arthralgia, fever, abdominal pain, clumsiness [Sydenham Chorea]	Probable acute rheumatic fever
Upper airway obstruction [snoring, marked difficulty breathing on an upper airway basis]	Possible prelude to Cor Pulmonale; look for early ECG changes such as right axis deviation, right atrial abnormality, prominent anterior or rightward forces for age
Congenital nerve deafness [Jervell-Lange-Nielsen]	Possible sudden death from ventricular arrhythmia associated with prolonged QTc interval on ECG [>.425 secs]; such patients may also present with apparent seizure disorders

Table 2.1: (Continued)

History or Observation	Correlation
High dietary salt intake	Possible hyperdynamic circulation with prominent precordial impulse, prominent peripheral pulses, S3, diastolic overload on ECG; especially important with family history of hypertension
IMPORTANT PERINATAL HISTORY	
Maternal Lupus Erythematosis	Possible congenital complete A-V block in the infant
Maternal exposure to viral agent or drug	Possible cardiac sequelae [see Table 1.2]
Maternal gestational diabetes	Possible congenital cardiac defect; possible neonatal transient cardiomyopathy; serum calcium and glucose levels may be low
Prematurity	Patent ductus arteriosus
Neonatal asphyxia [meconium aspiration] with hypoglycemia, hypocalcemia, and/or polycythemia	Possible persistent pulmonary hypertension [persistent fetal circulation]
IMPORTANT FAMILY CARDIOVASCULAR HISTORY	
First degree male relative less than 50 years old or female less than 60 years old with myocardial infarction	Familial hyperlipoproteinemia occurs in about 33% of families with such histories; consider screening with a 12 hour fasting serum cholesterol and triglyceride level

Table 2.1: (Continued)

History or Observation	Correlation
First degree relative with hypertension	Hypertension is often familial; careful BP monitoring and consideration of dietary salt restriction are necessary
Family history of palpitations	Cardiac arrhythmias are often familial

Table 2.2: Important Physical Finding Correlations

Physical Finding	Correlation
GENERAL APPEARANCE AND INSPECTION INCLUDING EVIDENCE FOR A GENETIC DISORDER	
Tall patient or patient with straight back, narrow thoracic A-P diameter, pectus excavatum, or scoliosis	High incidence of mitral valve prolapse [MVP] and/or tricuspid valve prolapse; as many as 16% females have MVP; listen for a systolic click; the tall patient may have Marfan syndrome which is also associated with a high incidence of MVP
Down Syndrome	High association of congenital cardiac defects [see Table 1.4 for other syndromes]
Tall, very slender infant or infant that appears almost cachectic	Consider chronic significant CHF
Fretful, irritable infant who is diaphoretic, grunting, dyspneic, pale or cyanotic	Classical findings of CHF which usually includes the triad of tachypnea, tachycardia and cardiomegaly
PALPATION	
Suprasternal Notch Thrill	Possible aortic or pulmonic stenosis; possible aortic coarctation or PDA
Systolic thrill at lower left sternal border	Probable VSD
Systolic thrill at upper left or upper right sternal border	Probable pulmonic or aortic stenosis, respectively

Table 2.2: (Continued)

Physical Finding	Correlation
Loss of sharp hepatic edge [i.e. rounded liver edge] even without overt hepatomegaly	Consider low grade, chronic CHF
Weak or absent femoral pulses or radial-femoral lag	Probable aortic coarctation
Unilateral decrease in upper extremity pulse	Consider aortic arch anomaly with stenosis of the subclavian artery origin
Bounding, symmetrical peripheral pulses	Consider PDA in infant and young child; consider aortic insufficiency in older child; consider hyperdynamic circulation associated with increased salt intake in older child
Pulses Bisferens	Probable hypertrophic obstructive cardiomyopathy
PRECORDIAL CARDIAC PALPATION	
Hyperdynamic apical impulse	Probable left to right shunt at ventricular or PDA level
Lateral displacement of apical impulse	Evidence for cardiomegaly
RV heave at lower left sternal border	Consider ASD or pulmonary hypertension

Table 2.2: (Continued)

Physical Finding	Correlation
CARDIAC AUSCULTATION	
Increased first heart sound [S1]	Consider short PR interval [pre-excitation syndrome such as Wolf-Parkinson-White]; consider endocardial cushion defect
Decreased S1	Consider first degree A-V block; may be obscured by holosystolic VSD murmur; if all heart sounds are decreased and have a "pitter-patter" quality consider cardiomyopathy or myocarditis with associated marked decrease in cardiac function
Single second heart sound [S2] with no accentuation	Consider missing semi-lunar valve such as in pulmonary atresia or aortic atresia; consider tetralogy of Fallot
Loud, single S2	Consider truncus arteriosus, transposition complex [complete transposition in cyanotic infant]; may represent a narrowly split S2 from extreme pulmonary hypertension
Narrowly split S2 with accentuated pulmonary component	Typical finding of pulmonary hypertension, usually secondary to large VSD
Prominently split S2 with no respiratory variation even in a sitting position	Classical finding of ASD or hemi-anomalous pulmonary venous return

Table 2.2: (Continued)

Physical Finding	Correlation
Presence of a third heart sound [S3]	Usually normal; if not previously present may represent CHF or hyperdynamic circulation
Presence of a fourth heart sound [S4]	Consider cardiomyopathy or other cause of difficulty filling the ventricles such as in severe aortic or pulmonic stenosis, or aortic coarctation
Systolic ejection click [early systolic click]	Consider mild to moderate aortic or pulmonic stenosis; consider isolated bicuspid aortic valve [6% of normal population]; if present between the apex and lower left sternal border, probable mitral or tricuspid valve prolapse; possible transient VSD aneurysm if present at mid left sternal border after disappearance of VSD murmur
Mid systolic click or clicks	Classical mitral valve prolapse
THE CARDIAC MURMURS	
Short, purely vibratory systolic ejection murmur along left sternal border, which usually changes intensity with positional changes	Classical innocent Still's murmur; if there are any harsh overtones, consider covert cardiomyopathy

Table 2.2: (Continued)

Physical Finding	Correlation
Harsh, basal systolic ejection murmurs	Probable aortic stenosis [upper right sternal border with superior radiation] or pulmonary stenosis [upper left sternal border].
Continuous, machinery quality or "rocky" murmur maximal in the left infra-clavicular area with some inferior or medial radiation; present in all positions	Classical significant PDA murmur; if the PDA is small then only a short, harsh, distinct systolic ejection murmur is present in the left infraclavicular area with usual radiation to the back
Raspy, long, holosystolic murmur maximal at the lower left sternal border	Classical VSD murmur
Non-specific, slightly harsh systolic ejection murmur at mid left sternal border associated with systolic click and single diminished second heart sound	Usual findings of tetralogy of Fallot [click is from aortic dilatation; murmur represents forward flow across the stenotic pulmonary outflow region, not the right to left ventricular shunt flow]
Decrescendo, early, high pitched, blowing, echoing diastolic murmur along aortic ejection path between upper right sternal border and apex	Classical aortic insufficiency murmur; carefully search for this murmur in children with VSD because subaortic VSD may be associated with aortic insufficiency
Similar quality murmur but maximal over pulmonary valve area	Pulmonary insufficiency; often present after repair of tetralogy of Fallot

Table 2.2: (Continued)

Physical Finding	Correlation
Blowing long systolic apical murmur radiating to left axilla	Probable mitral insufficiency [not common in children other than in association with endocardial cushion defects]
Apical systolic whoop or honk	Unusual form of murmurs associated with mitral valve prolapse [probably represents minimal mitral insufficiency]; may be loud enough to hear without stethoscope
Short, harsh systolic ejection murmur, maximal over pulmonary area with distinct lateral radiation to both axillae and to back, in an infant or child less than eighteen months of age	Typical description of physiological peripheral pulmonary stenosis; this usually disappears by 18 to 24 months of age; if such a murmur persists beyond 24 months of age, consider true anatomical peripheral pulmonary stenosis
Continuous, roaring murmur in either infraclavicular area present only with the child sitting. External pressure over the jugular regions, change in neck position, and assuming a reclining position usually obliterates the murmur.	Classical benign venous hum; note disappearance upon the patient reclining

Chapter 3

Non-Invasive Diagnostic Aids

Remarkable advances in non-invasive diagnostic procedures occurred during the past five years. Two-dimensional [real time or cross sectional] echocardiography now enhanced by Doppler analysis allows very accurate determination of intracardiac and great vessel anatomy. Doppler evaluation is able to accurately determine physiological data such as instantaneous pressure differences across semi-lunar and A-V valves. Magnetic Resonance Imaging [MRI] adds another perspective to anatomical definition, but more importantly will likely enable assessment of myocardial metabolic states, using very high energy magnetic fields [magnetic resonance spectroscopy or MRS]. The result of our newer technologies is a reduction in the number of invasive procedures such as diagnostic cardiac catheterization. Interventional cardiac catheterization such as balloon dilation of pulmonary or aortic stenosis often replaces the purely diagnostic cath procedures. Furthermore, with advances in surgery allowing total repair of complex congenital heart defects at very early ages, the need to assess precise cardiac physiology, such as pulmonary vascular resistance, is much less important.

This chapter will outline the major non-invasive techniques, including ECG and chest radiographs, as well as the exciting new capabilities.

THE PEDIATRIC ECG

Pediatric House Officer interpretation of the pediatric ECG is often fraught with extreme anxiety and therefore resisted. Using a very simple approach to ECG interpretation, the author hopes to convey a sense of understanding of the pediatric ECG that will allow house officers to accurately and confidently determine major ECG abnormalities in pediatric patients.

The most important notion is that electrical vectors traveling toward a positively referenced electrode result in positive deflections and those traveling away from a positively referenced electrode result in negative deflections. If a vector is perpendicular to the reference electrode, the net deflection of that electrode's recording will approach 0 and we refer to such a waveform on the ECG as isoelectric or nearly isoelectric. These concepts are true whether we speak of P waves, QRS deflections, or T waves. Figure 3.1 reviews these vector concepts. Figure 3.2 presents the classical hexagonal representation of the frontal ECG leads, labeling the leads where they are positive by convention. Conceptually, one is viewing the frontal plane ECG vectors from each of these different perspectives upon switching from frontal lead to frontal lead on the actual ECG machine. It is as though we were viewing objects within a given square room from several different windows around the room. After some study of this hexagonal labeling system one should realize that there are three perpendicular lead sets: Leads I and AVF, Leads AVL and II, Leads AVR and III are 90 degrees apart.

Frontal QRS Axis: Using the concept that an isoelectric waveform identifies the lead that is perpendicular to the true frontal vector, one can usually estimate the frontal axis. For example if the isoelectric waveform was identified in Lead AVR as is often true in the neonate, when the RV is relatively dominant, then the frontal vector would be along lead III [the perpendicular to AVR] at +120, also assuming that the waveform in this lead was positive. Certainly the perpendicular to a given lead can be 90 degrees away in either direction, for which reason one has to scan the frontal leads in the region of interest and determine which 90 degree direction the frontal vector truly points. Most discussions on determination of the frontal QRS vector summarize methods to at least determine in which quadrant the frontal vector rests. With a slightly greater effort, one can estimate the direction of the frontal vector with even greater accuracy. The additional information required is the fact that a lead may not be exactly isoelectric but still allow estimation of the frontal vector. If a lead is mostly isoelectric and yet slightly positive, overall, then the frontal vector is slightly closer to that reference lead and less than 90 degrees away. Similarly if the most isoelectric lead is slightly negative, overall, then the true frontal vector

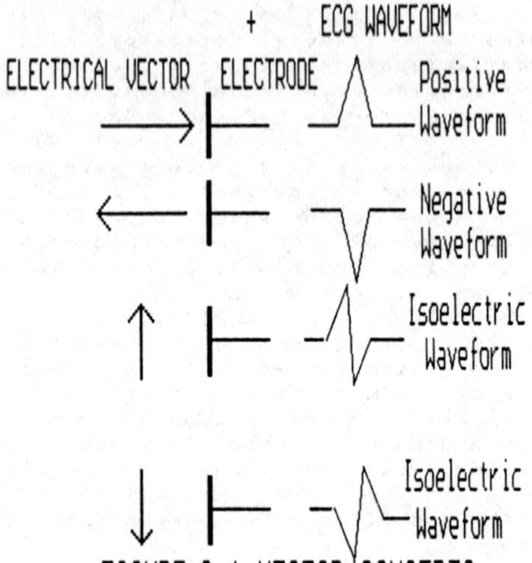

FIGURE 3.1:VECTOR CONCEPTS

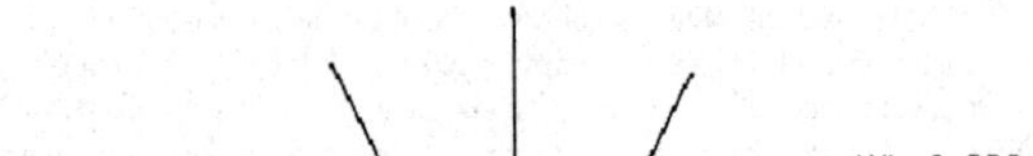

FIGURE 3.2: FRONTAL ECG LEADS

is slightly further from that reference lead or slightly greater than 90 degrees away. As an example assume that lead AVL is most isoelectric but also slightly negative, overall [the negative deflection exceeds the positive deflection, slightly]. If AVL were exactly isoelectric then the frontal vector would be +60 degrees, assuming Lead II were positive. With AVL slightly more negative than positive, the true frontal vector is slightly more than 90 degrees away from AVL and possibly another 10 to 15 degrees away or at approximately 70 to 75 degrees.

Table 3.1 estimates the frontal QRS axis using the above concepts. In order to estimate the frontal axis, choose the most isoelectric lead on a given ECG. Then decide whether the perpendicular lead is negative or positive. Determine whether the isoelectric lead appears slightly more positive, slightly more negative, or exactly isoelectric. Note the estimated axis along the appropriate column.

Significance of Frontal QRS Axis: Although right axis deviation for age suggests RV dominance and left axis deviation for age suggests LV dominance, one of the more important findings relating to a possible serious congenital cardiac malformation is the discovery of a *superior QRS axis.* Pediatric cardiologists have classically referred to left axis deviation greater than -30 degrees as *Left Superior Axis*. In most cases, the finding is an indication of left anterior hemi-block and this frontal axis is associated with the following serious congenital heart defects:

ACYANOTIC:

1. Endocardial Cushion Defect [spectrum includes Ostium Primum ASD to Complete Atrio-Ventricular Canal]
2. Double outlet RV with sub-pulmonary VSD [these patients may be slightly desaturated, systemically].

CYANOTIC:

1. Tricuspid Atresia Complex with Normally Related Great Vessels
2. Complete Transposition [D-Loop/D-Transposition] with associated VSD
3. Double Outlet RV with sub-aortic VSD [Taussig-Bing Anomaly].

The finding of a left superior QRS axis may be the only clue that a newborn with Down Syndrome has a significant congenital cardiac defect. In the postoperative state, such a finding indicates left anterior hemi-block, if the finding was not present, pre-operatively. In this situation, if there is an associated complete right bundle

Table 3.1: Determination of Frontal QRS Axis

MOST ISOELECTRIC LEAD [AXIS]	IS WAVEFORM IN PERPENDICULAR LEAD POSITIVE OR NEGATIVE?	IS ISOELECTRIC LEAD MORE POSITIVE OR NEGATIVE?	ESTIMATED FRONTAL AXIS
I [0]	AVF [+90]	NEITHER	+ 90
I	IS	POSITIVE	+ 75
I	POSITIVE	NEGATIVE	+105
I [0]	AVF [+90]	NEITHER	- 90
I	IS	POSITIVE	- 75
I	NEGATIVE	NEGATIVE	-105
II [+60]	AVL [-30]	NEITHER	+150
II	IS	POSITIVE	+135
II	NEGATIVE	NEGATIVE	+165
II [+60]	AVL [-30]	NEITHER	-30
II	IS	POSITIVE	-15
II	POSITIVE	NEGATIVE	-45
III [+120]	AVR [+30]	NEITHER	+30
III	IS	POSITIVE	+45
III	NEGATIVE	NEGATIVE	+15
III [+120]	AVR [+30]	NEITHER	-150
III	IS	POSITIVE	-165
III	POSITIVE	NEGATIVE	-135
AVR [-150]	III [+120]	NEITHER	+120
AVR	IS	POSITIVE	+135
AVR	POSITIVE	NEGATIVE	+105
AVR [-150]	III [+120]	NEITHER	- 60
AVR	IS	POSITIVE	- 75
AVR	NEGATIVE	NEGATIVE	- 45
AVL [-30]	II [+60]	NEITHER	+ 60
AVL	IS	POSITIVE	+ 45
AVL	POSITIVE	NEGATIVE	+ 75
AVL [-30]	II [+60]	NEITHER	-120
AVL	IS	POSITIVE	-105
AVL	NEGATIVE	NEGATIVE	-135
AVF [+90]	I [0]	NEITHER	0
AVF	IS	POSITIVE	+15
AVF	POSITIVE	NEGATIVE	-15
AVF [+90]	I [0]	NEITHER	+/-180
AVF	IS	POSITIVE	+165
AVF	NEGATIVE	NEGATIVE	-165

branch block, the child would have bi-fascicular disease and there would be a higher risk of sudden death. Electrophysiological studies may determine the risk of sudden catastrophe more accurately, in such patients.

Right superior axis [-90 to -180 degrees] may have the same significance as left superior axis in a given child. If all leads on an ECG are essentially iso-electric, then the frontal axis would be *Indeterminate.* This finding also suggests one of the lesions listed under left superior QRS axis, and indicates electrically, that there is a broad frontal QRS loop with the major axis pointing either directly anteriorly or posteriorly.

Along with frontal QRS estimate, the house officer should be able to assess the basic ECG rhythm in a given child. There is no room for discussions of complex arrhythmias but if the house officer is familiar with what is usually normal in children, significant deviation from the normal rhythm would be detected. The basic five rhythms in children are:

1. Normal Sinus Rhythm where there is a steady rate with little R-R interval variation. Each QRS complex would have a preceding P wave.

2. Normal Sinus Arrhythmia where there is slight rhythm variation related directly to breathing in that inspiration causes a slight increase in heart rate and the beginning of expiration is associated with a slight decrease in heart rate. This phenomenon relates to normal vagal tone in children.

3. Prominent Sinus Arrhythmia where there is considerable rate variation, but this variation still relates to breathing. Associated with this finding is the benign wandering atrial pacemaker, indicated by subtle change in P wave morphology in a rhythmic pattern as well. During periods of slow rate it is common for the pacemaker to shift to a lower focus and therefore for the P waves to become inverted in the inferior leads II, III, AVF. Actually, the finding of a constant low right atrial pacemaker in a child [P waves constantly inverted in inferior leads II, III, AVF and positive in lead I] is usually felt to be normal variation and benign. One should be aware of the fact that in children with increased intracranial pressure [e.g., secondary to meningitis], there is often an associated wandering pacemaker.

4. Sinus Tachycardia where heart rate exceeds the normal range for age [see Tables 3.2/3.3 Normal Pediatric ECG Values]. One should be aware of the fact that sinus

tachycardia may be as high as 200 BPM in agitated children or children with high fevers. Rates over 200 BPM suggest paroxysmal supraventricular tachycardia or other supraventricular dysrhythmia.

5. Sinus Bradycardia where heart rate is lower than expected for age [see Tables 3.2/3.3]. This may be benign in the well trained athlete. However, bradycardia in the neonate is usually significant and requires immediate evaluation. The newborn may tolerate complete heart block well, but cardiology evaluation is very important. In such a case, there would be no constant relationship between P waves and the QRS complexes. The atrial rate would be normal for age, whereas the ventricular rate would be very decreased, if complete heart block were present.

<u>The Intervals [PR/ QRS/ QTc]</u>: After determination of rhythm and frontal QRS axis, the next logical step in ECG interpretation is measurement of the important intervals

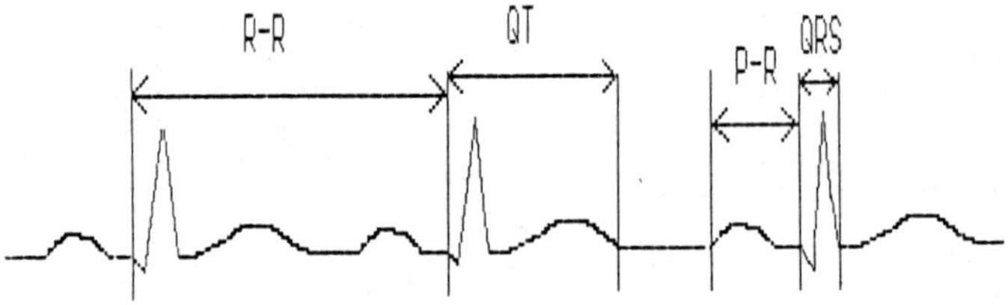

$$QTc = QT/\sqrt{R\text{-}R\ [Preceding]}$$

NORMAL QTc = .38 - .425 [.44] sec

<u>FIGURE 3.3: ECG INTERVALS</u>

[see Fig. 3.3]. It is very important to calculate a corrected QTc interval so that one may make an accurate determination of shortening or prolongation relative to heart rate at any age.

PR Interval: The PR interval is either normal, prolonged, or shortened, according to age and heart rate. It is important to relate heart rate and age to PR interval. PR interval prolongation reflects a First Degree A-V Block and may be associated with the following:

1. Normal variant, possibly even familial variant.

2. About 10% of children with uncomplicated ASD, VSD have first degree A-V Block.

3. This finding is common in children with Endocardial Cushion Defect whether it represents Ostium Primum ASD or Complete A-V Canal.

4. Acute Rheumatic Fever [ARF] is associated with this ECG finding as a minor criterion. It does not reflect myocarditis and in fact one book on ARF stated that 10% of children with uncomplicated Group A Streptococcal pharyngitis develop a transient First Degree A-V Block.

5. In only one major instance is PR interval prolongation somewhat ominous and possibly reflects progression to second degree and then complete heart block. This involves patients with otherwise uncomplicated *Corrected Transposition [L-Loop, L-Transposition]*. This entity basically involves anatomical ventricular inversion. Even if no other intracardiac defects are present in a given patient with this malformation, there is a progressive tendency toward the development of higher degrees of A-V Block, starting with first degree block. Such patients often require permanent pacemaker placement.

Short PR interval could be a reflection of pre-excitation conduction such as Wolff-Parkinson-White or Lown-Ganong-Levine. In the first case prominent delta waves are present and in the latter case, normal QRS morphology is present with the short PR interval. Figures 3.4 and 3.5 demonstrate these concepts. Patients with either form of pre-excitation often have recurrent supraventricular tachycardias that may require therapy. Children with Glycogen Storage Disease [associated with large tongues], may have a short PR interval on the ECG because glycogen is an excellent electrical conductor.

Physical exam may reflect the PR interval in that a *prolonged PR interval* is often associated with a *diminished first heart sound*, whereas a *short PR interval* is often associated with an *increased first heart sound*. In the first instance, more time is allowed for the A-V valves to

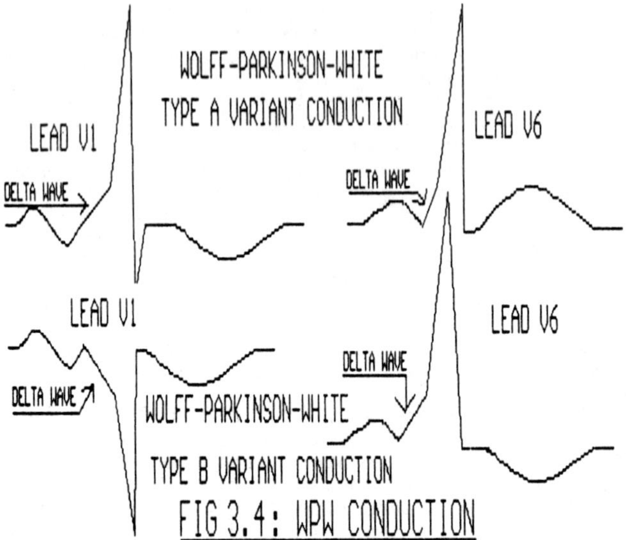

FIG 3.4: WPW CONDUCTION

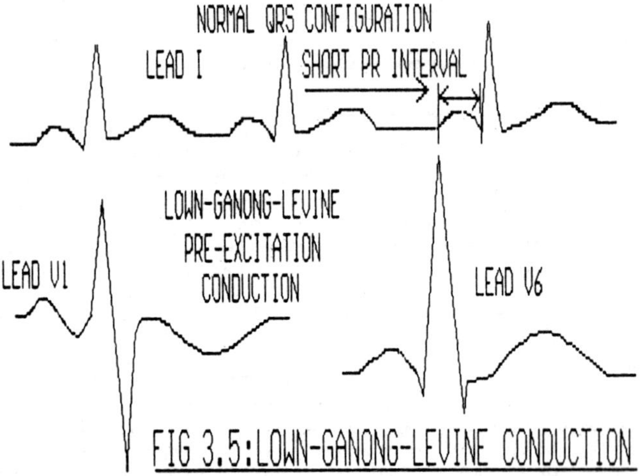

FIG 3.5:LOWN-GANONG-LEVINE CONDUCTION

float back to a more closed position, resulting in a diminished intensity of S1; with short PR interval, the A-V valves are widely separated during early isovolumic contraction, resulting in an increased S1.

QRS Duration: Prolongation of the QRS interval reflects one of three possibilities, in general terms:

1. Complete Right Bundle Branch Block [CRBBB]
2. Complete Left Bundle Branch Block [CLBBB]
3. Intraventricular Conduction Block [IVCB].

Typical waveforms for Right and Left Bundle Branch Blocks appear in Figure 3.6. When the QRS duration is prolonged and the precordial waveforms do not conform to either Right or Left Bundle Branch Block, then an Intraventricular Conduction Block is likely present. Severe myocardial dysfunction or damage may be associated with this form of QRS prolongation. CLBBB is rare in children whereas CRBBB is not uncommon, either congenitally or especially after surgical correction of lesions such as large VSD or tetralogy of Fallot. If unassociated with First Degree A-V Block or left anterior hemi-block, CRBBB is usually quite benign.

Importantly, an ECG that demonstrates right bundle branch morphology with *normal QRS duration*, actually reflects an intraventricular conduction delay, consistent with diastolic overload as one would have with atrial septal defect. However if the R′ waveform is less than 5 mm on normal standard tracing, then the configuration represents a normal intraventricular conduction delay and is less suggestive of diastolic overload. Also with diastolic overload associated with atrial septal defect, rightward forces are usually increased as well. Figure 3.7 demonstrates these concepts.

QTc Interval: The corrected QT interval should be within a normal range of .38 to .425 sec or 380 to 425 msec regardless of age or heart rate. Values between .425 and .44 seconds would be borderline prolongation, and any values over .44 seconds would be significantly prolonged. Determination of QTc interval involves measurement of a QT interval [onset of Q or R wave to end of T wave] on one of the frontal leads with best QRS-T definition and dividing this value by the square root of the preceding R-R interval [see Figure 3.3]. Generally one would want to choose the area of the tracing with the shortest R-R intervals to maximize the QTc calculation and therefore to avoid missing

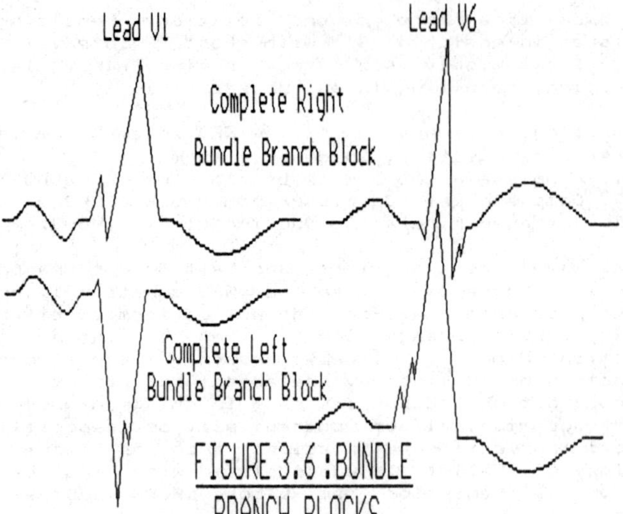

FIGURE 3.6 : BUNDLE BRANCH BLOCKS

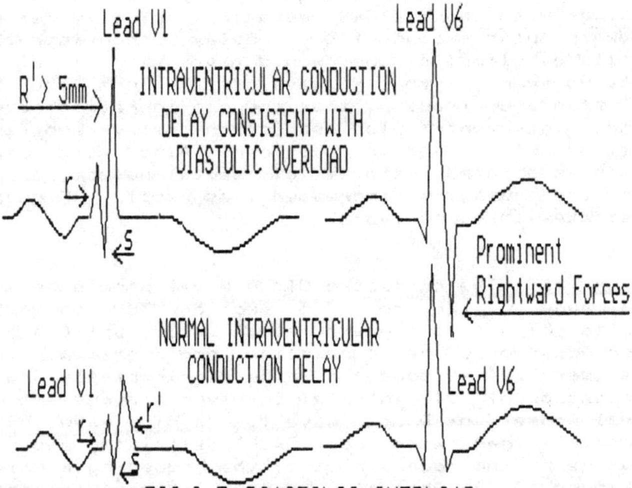

FIG 3.7 : DIASTOLIC OVERLOAD

a prolonged QTc interval. One usually makes several calculations for comparison. If the frontal leads do not permit good definition of the QRS-T waves, then a precordial lead may be chosen, with the understanding that this calculation is likely not as accurate on the precordial leads. The calculation is also not perfect, and one observes considerable QTc variation in children with prominent sinus arrhythmias.

QTc prolongation occurs:

1. In patients with a *decreased ionized calcium* [especially true in the neonate or after administration of large amounts of base such as sodium bicarbonate in a child that had metabolic acidosis]

2. After administration of certain beta 2 agents such as *metaproterenol* or *terbutaline*

3. After administration of anti-arrhythmic agents such as *Quinidine* or *Norpace* (disopyramide *phosphate*)

4. In possible association with *idiopathic prolonged QT interval syndrome*. This latter association is the most dangerous and least well understood. Sympathetic imbalance of the stellate ganglia is likely involved with QTc prolongation in patients who are at risk of sudden death from recurrent ventricular tachycardia. In such cases, the ventricular tachycardia may become ventricular fibrillation and cause syncope followed by sudden death. Syncope in such patients is ominous and one should at least try phenytoin or propranolol to control syncopal episodes in such children. Agents such as Norpace are contraindicated in these patients. Rarely sympathectomy has been used to control arrhythmias in these instances. Exercise or vagal maneuvers may be necessary to uncover QTc prolongation in any one patient.

Shortening of the QTc interval is associated with:

1. Digoxin administration

2. Increased serum *ionized* calcium [as occurs with metabolic or respiratory acidemia]

3. Occasionally after administration of beta 2 agents as noted above.

P wave morphology: Frontal P waves are usually positive in the inferior leads when a child is in normal sinus rhythm. As noted above, it is quite common for children to manifest low right atrial rhythm in which case the frontal P waves are flat or inverted in the inferior leads II, III, AVF. Apart from the P wave vector, observation of the P wave morphology can suggest right and/or left atrial abnormality [see Fig. 3.8]. The author uses the term *abnormality* to indicate that one cannot differentiate between hypertrophy and acute dilation of the atria, electrocardiographically. *Tall, peaked P waves* exceeding 2.5 to 3 mm. deflection, suggest *right atrial abnormality* [Fig. 3.8]. This finding is quite common in congenital cardiac defects resulting in RV hypertension or poorly compliant RV [e.g., severe pulmonary stenosis, tetralogy of Fallot] or in Tricuspid Atresia complexes. Early Cor Pulmonale [RV failure] from upper airway obstruction is also associated with this ECG finding. *Prolongation of the frontal P wave duration beyond .10 sec suggests left atrial abnormality* [Fig. 3.8]. Left atrial abnormality is also often suggested on the precordial leads V1/V4R if the P waves in these leads are biphasic and the posterior [negative] component exceeds 1 mm. x 1 mm. deflections. Lesions that result in increased

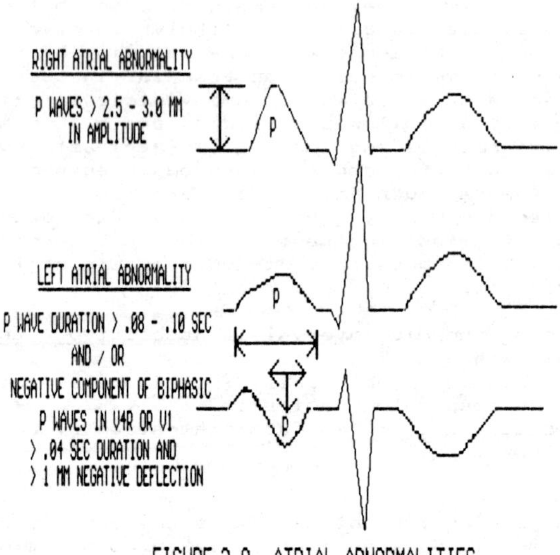

FIGURE 3.8: ATRIAL ABNORMALITIES

LA flow such as VSD or PDA or that result in difficulty filling the LV such as severe aortic stenosis or cardiomyopathy, often reflect LA abnormality on the ECG. The author has noted that pectus excavatum and narrow thoracic Anterior-Posterior [AP] diameter are also associated with this finding, as is obesity.

T wave morphology: Once familiar with standard, normal ECG tracings, the house officer will be comfortable with normal T wave morphology. The most common normal variant that leads to concern is early T wave repolarization which results in tall T waves throughout the ECG, especially on the precordial leads. Often one is able to identify the "glitch" immediately after the QRS waveform connecting such a T wave. The only other significant cause for such T waves would be hyperkalemia, which could certainly be determined by lab test, if a true concern arose. Flat or inverted T waves are present with hypokalemia, but in general the author shuns use of the ECG for electrolyte monitoring because such changes are not consistent and they reflect large deflections from normal serum electrolyte levels.

Myocarditis, cardiomyopathy, and extreme forms of congenital heart disease resulting in severe CHF may all be associated with severe ST-T wave abnormalities, reflecting myocardial ischemia or dysfunction.

Interesting and unexplained T wave changes occur in about 50% of patients with mitral valve prolapse where T waves in Lead III are often inverted and those in leads II, AVF, V5, and V6 are flat or inverted. Such findings also occur in patients taking Beta 2 agents such as metaproterenol or terbutaline [see under QTc interval as well]. The highly trained athlete such as professional football player also has similar inferior T wave changes (1). The author has discovered that such T wave changes are often uncovered when the child is asked to sit. The sitting ECG may show such inferior and/or lateral T wave changes whereas the reclining tracing could be normal.

Ordinarily the QRS and T waves are concordant in a given lead [i.e., their vectors are in the same general direction, with both upright or both inverted]. In cases where they are discordant, one is often dealing with a wide QRS-T angle and this may be evidence for global myocardial dysfunction [see intraventricular conduction block above, also].

The Assessment of Ventricular Hypertrophies: One of the most confusing problems of ECG interpretation appears to be evaluation of ventricular hypertrophy. With a few basic principles the house officer should be able to determine whether major hypertrophy problems exist. The author tries to avoid tables adding two lead voltages, and would rather concentrate upon what ventricle the various waveforms usually reflect on the precordial leads. For simplicity, discussions pertaining to ventricular hypertrophy will involve precordial Leads V4R/V1 and V5/V6, apart from biventricular hypertrophy when mid precordial leads V3/V4 are involved. Using Figure 3.9 for reference, it should become apparent that leads V4R and V1 reflect anterior and posterior forces. Anterior forces are R waves in these leads whereas posterior forces are S waves in these leads.

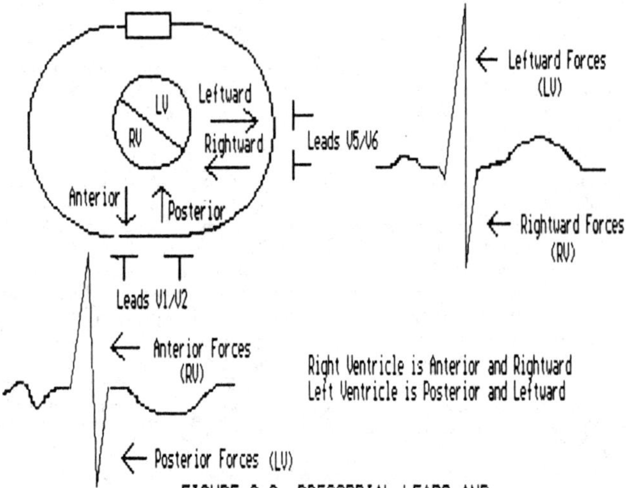

FIGURE 3.9: PRECORDIAL LEADS AND VENTRICULAR HYPERTROPHY

Similarly, leads V5/V6 reflect leftward and rightward forces. Leftward forces are R waves in these leads whereas rightward forces are S waves in these leads. Understanding that the RV is anterior and to the right, it makes sense that RVH reflects an increase in anterior [R waves V4R/V1] and rightward [S waves V5/V6] forces; LVH reflects an increase in posterior [S waves V4R/V1] and leftward forces [R waves in V5/V6] Tables are available for limits of R wave and S wave amplitude in these standard leads. Even if the house officer is uncertain about absolute evidence for ventricular hypertrophy, it is perfectly reasonable to conclude that increased rightward or increased leftward forces for age exist in a given child, without indicating overt RVH or LVH. At least one may identify a possible problem with one or other ventricle. Besides obvious increases in the above waveform amplitudes there are certain principles associated with ventricular hypertrophy that do not conform to the simple notion of increased precordial forces.

RVH: 1. Pure R waves in leads V4R or V1. One must differentiate this finding from a nearly pure R wave as a result of an intraventricular conduction delay [e.g., RR′]. Pediatric tracings include lead V4R because this lead gives another electrical window to the Right Ventricle, which is often involved in many congenital cardiac defects.

2. A qR waveform in leads V4R or V1. In cases of Corrected Transposition this waveform may reflect ventricular inversion in lieu of ventricular hypertrophy. In this instance one often finds no septal q waves in the left precordial leads V5/V6. Remember that the septum depolarizes from left to right in the normal heart, resulting in a small septal q wave in the lateral leads. With ventricular inversion, septal depolarization occurs from right to left and therefore, the initial deflection is toward the lateral leads V5/V6, blending with the R wave in those leads. At the same time this septal depolarization is moving away from the anterior and rightward leads V4R/V1, resulting in a q wave in those leads.

3. Upright T waves in leads V4R/V1 in children between the ages of 3 days to about 8 years old, are evidence alone of significant RVH. The reason for this is not completely known, but this is an important finding. In the immediate newborn period [0-72 hours], T waves may normally be upright in leads V4R/V1, so that one needs to repeat a tracing done in this age group, if T waves are truly upright in these leads. It is also important to make certain that T waves in the rest of the tracing appear normal. For example, with myocarditis, T waves may be

inverted in most leads, in which case one cannot conclude that an upright T wave in leads V4R/V1 reflect RVH.

LVH: Apart from absolute increases in posterior and leftward forces, the following two findings may suggest mild left ventricular prominence without overt hypertrophy:

1. Flat inferior and/or lateral ST segments
2. R wave amplitudes in lead V6 that are equal to or greater than R wave amplitudes in lead V5, even though they may not exceed normals for age. This finding is not found in textbooks, and is the author's personal observation. The author does not believe that it is normal for R wave amplitudes in lead V6 to exceed those in lead V5. In one child followed by the author, the only suggestion of LV dominance or an LV problem was the finding of a greater R wave amplitude in lead V6 compared with V5. The patient was later followed and found to have obstructive hypertrophic cardiomyopathy with overt LVH later in his course.

Biventricular hypertrophy [BVH]: An adult ECG criterion for BVH involves equiphasic mid precordial voltages that exceed 50 mm. in amplitude. In children this is not an uncommon normal finding and one suspects BVH only if mid precordial voltages exceed 60-70 mm. in amplitude. Certainly if a child has evidence for overt RVH [e.g., pure R wave V4R/V1] and also has leftward forces that are increased for age, one could conclude that BVH exists.

TABLE 3.2: PEDIATRIC ECG NORMAL VALUES
[BIRTH TO 6 MONTHS] (1)

	[- - - - - -AGE IN DAYS			- - - - - -]	[AGE IN MONTHS]	
	0-1	1-3	3-7	7-30	1-3	3-6
HR (2)	99-148	97-149	100-161	114-178	124-175	112-178
QRS AXIS	92-185	94-186	92-185	78-151	46-105	18-93
PR [secs]	.08-.14	.09-.13	.08-.13	.08-.13	.08-.13	.08-.14
PR [secs] (3,4)	.07-.12	.07-.12	.07-.12	.07-.11	.07-.13	.07-.13
QRS [secs]	.03-.07	.03-.06	.03-.06	.03-.08	.03-.07	.03-.08
P LEAD II[mm]	.5-2.5	.5-2.5	1-2.5	1-3	1-2	1-2.5
V1 R [mm]	7-24	5-24	5-21	4-19	5-17	5-17
V1 S [mm]	1-18	2-19	1-15	1-10	1-11	1-13
V5 R [mm]	3-19	4-20	5-19	6-21	11-29	13-32
V5 S [mm]	4-18	2-16	4-17	3-14	3-13	2-15
V6 R [mm]	2-9	1-10	1-10	3-14	6-19	8-20
V6 S [mm]	0-8	0-8	1-8	1-8	1-6	0-7
V3R R [mm]	4-18	5-20	2-18	3-15	3-12	2-11
V3R S [mm]	1-12	1-12	1-8	0-5	0-6	1-8
R/S V3R	.3-4.6	.4-4.3	.2-5.2	.5-4.5	.2-4.5	.1-2.3
R/S V1	.4-7	.4-5.4	.5-7.4	1.2-6.4	.7-5.9	.3-5.6
R+S V4 [mm]	16-47	20-48	17-44	18-44	25-50	25-56
RV6+SV1 [mm]	3-24	4-25	4-22	4-19	8-26	10-32

V4R data (5,6)

AGE:	30 hrs	1 mo	2-3 mo	4-5 mo
R [mm]	4-14	3-9	1-10	2-8
S [mm]	0-13	1-5	0-9	0-7

QTc interval should be between .38 and .425 seconds. Values over .44 seconds are significantly prolonged.

TABLE 3.3: PEDIATRIC ECG NORMAL VALUES [6 MONTHS TO 16 YEARS] (1)

[AGE IN MONTHS]	[- - - - - - -AGE IN YEARS- - - - - - - -]					
	6-12	1-3	3-5	5-8	8-12	12-16
HR (2)	112-163	97-144	81-132	72-126	66-124	64-114
QRS AXIS	16-87	18-90	15-88	21-106	19-101	19-111
PR [secs]	.08-.14	.09-.14	.09-.15	.09-.16	.09-.17	.10-.17
PR [secs] (3,4)	.08-.13	.08-.15	.09-.15	.10-.16	.10-.17	.11-.16
QRS [secs]	.03-.07	.03-.07	.03-.07	.04-.08	.04-.08	.04-.08
P LEAD II[mm]	1-2.5	1-2.5	.5-2.5	.5-2.5	.5-2.5	.5-2.5
V1 R [mm]	3-17	3-15	3-15	2-12	1-11	1-9
V1 S [mm]	1-14	2-18	3-19	4-21	4-21	4-19
V5 R [mm]	12-29	11-29	13-34	16-38	16-37	11-33
V5 S [mm]	1-13	1-10	1-9	1-9	1-7	1-6
V6 R [mm]	7-19	8-20	9-22	10-24	11-24	8-21
V6 S [mm]	0-6	0-5	0-4	0-4	0-4	0-3
V3R R [mm]	1-11	2-10	2-9	1-9	1-8	1-6
V3R S [mm]	1-8	1-11	2-12	2-13	2-15	2-13
R/S V3R	.1-1.9	0-1.4	0-.9	0-.7	0-.7	0-.7
R/S V1	.3-3.5	.2-3.4	.1-2	.1-1.7	.1-1.5	.1-1.2
R+S V4 [mm]	23-46	21-45	23-48	22-49	23-48	15-45
RV6+SV1 [mm]	10-29	10-34	15-38	16-41	17-42	15-37

V4R data (5,6)

AGE:	6-8 mo	9 mo-2 yr	2-5 yr	6-13 y
R [mm]	1-7	0-7	2-7	1-6
S [mm]	0-12	1-8	1-10	1-13

QTc interval should be between .38 and .425 seconds. Values over .44 seconds are significantly prolonged.

Importantly, the adult upper limit for PR interval is .20 sec. and for QRS duration is .10 sec..

Table 3.2 and 3.3 Notes

1. Modified from Davignon A, Rautaharju P, Boisselle E, Soumis F, Megelas M, Choquette A: Normal ECG Standards for Infants and Children. *Ped Cardiol* 1:123-152,1979/1980.

2. All data represents limits of 5th and 95th percentiles.

3. Liebman J, Plonsey R: Electrocardiography. In Moss A, Adams F, Emmanouilides G [eds]: *Heart Disease in Infants, Children, and Adolescents* [2nd edition]. Baltimore, Williams & Wilkins, 1977, p 31.

4. Ziegler RF: *Electrocardiographic Studies in Normal Infants and Children.* Springfield, Charles C Thomas, 1951.

5. Liebman J, Plonsey R: Electrocardiography. In Moss A, Adams F, Emmanouilides G [eds]: *Heart Disease in Infants, Children, and Adolescents* [2nd edition]. Baltimore, Williams & Wilkins, 1977, p 35.

6. Namin EP, Miller RA: The Normal Electrocardiogram and Vectorcardiogram in Children. In Cassels DE, Ziegler RF [eds]: *Electrocardiography in Infants and Children.* New York, Grune and Stratton, 1966, pp 99-115.

M-MODE ECHOCARDIOGRAPHIC DIMENSIONS AND FUNCTIONAL ESTIMATES IN INFANTS AND CHILDREN:

Introduction: With the advent of Real Time (2-D) echocardiographic imaging of infants and children, an entirely new ability to non-invasively assess complex congenital heart defects developed. Nevertheless, accurate ultrasound measurement of pediatric cardiac structures remains essential. During the early development of M-Mode pediatric echocardiography, many groups published their own sets of normal data using subtly different techniques of measurement. We have decided to present only one set of normal values that appears to have a unifying application to both children and adults, through regression equations based upon Age (yrs) and Body Surface Area (BSA [M^2]) or Age (yrs) and Weight (Kg) alone.

Standard pediatric cardiac dimensions: Concentrating upon the pediatric patient, it is apparent that standard cardiac dimensions change serially with growth. Whereas most early tables of normal echocardiographic values in children presented data grouped arbitrarily according to age and/or weight ranges, Walter L. Henry, M.D., et al (2), presented a series of useful regression equations that allowed calculation of standard dimensions as a continuum based upon Age and BSA or Age and Weight. In this group's study, a correlation coefficient (r) of 0.999 occurred upon relating BSA to Weight according to the equation: BSA = 0.12 x Weight(Kg)^.64 [^ = raised to the power of]. With this type of correlation, data did not vary significantly if one chose only weight compared with choosing BSA to derive normal values. The authors concluded that Weight alone was likely as accurate as using BSA in patients that were within 25% of standard Height and Weight, but could not comment upon accuracy differences in patients who were significantly outside the range of standard height and weight. The two tables below summarize the two sets of regression equations; 95% confidence limits are expressed as a percent of the value calculated for a given age and BSA or Weight. In our calculations the following equation is used to determine BSA [M^2] because it has application to both infants and adults (3):

BSA [M^2]= 0.024265 x H^.3964 x W^.5378.

H = Height(cm); W = Weight(kg); ^ = raised to the power of

Right Ventricular dimensions are not included because of the great variability and difficulty in standardizing this dimension. Henry used standards recommended by the American Society of Echocardiography (A.S.E.) to measure all dimensions (4).

BSA [M^2]/ Age [Years]/ Weight [KG]/ Dimensions [mm]

TABLE 3.4:

MEASUREMENTS (mm)	EQUATION
Aortic Root Dimension	24.0xBSA^(1/3)+0.1xAGE-4.3 +/-18%
Left Atrial Dimension	28.5xBSA^(1/3)+.08xAGE-0.9 +/-18%

LV End Diastolic Dimen	45.3xBSA^(1/3)-.03xAGE-7.2 +/-12%
LV End Systolic Dimen	28.8xBSA^(1/3)-.03xAGE-4.1 +/-18%
Septal Thickness	5.44xBSA^(1/2)+.03xAGE+1.5 +/-18%
LV Free Wall Thickness	5.56xBSA^(1/2)+.03xAGE+1.1 +/-16%

Table 3.5:

MEASUREMENTS	EQUATION
Aortic Root Dimension	11.8xWT^(.213)+0.1xAGE-4.3 +/-18%
Left Atrial Dimension	14.1xWT^(.213)+.08xAGE-0.9 +/-18%
LV End-Diastolic Dimen	22.4xWT^(.213)-.03xAGE-7.2 +/-12%
LV End-Systolic Dimen	14.2xWT^(.213)-.03xAGE-4.1 +/-18%
Septal Thickness	1.88xWT^(0.32)+.03xAGE+1.5 +/-18%
LV Free Wall Thickness	1.92xWT^(0.32)+.03xAGE+1.1 +/-16%

Left atrial dimension in early work [and in some labs presently], was measured from the posterior surface of the posterior aortic wall echo to the anterior surface of the posterior left atrial endocardium [inside dimensions of LA chamber]. This method will result in a smaller left atrial dimension compared with the A.S.E. measurement. When comparing data to normals, one must be absolutely certain as to the methods used for deriving the normal values. To promote uniformity and reproducibility one should make all measurements according to the A.S.E. standards. This should ensure that all future normal tables reflect similar measurements methods. For interest, there are at least three excellent books devoted solely to pediatric M-Mode echocardiography (4,5,6).Publication dates reflect the timing of this relatively old technology. In these texts one may find many other standard tables. Once again pay careful attention to the exact method of measurement.

Before ending this discussion of basic normal M-Mode dimensions one should mention the utility of Left Atrial/ Aortic Ratios. Specifically in Premature Infants, the presence of a Patent Ductus Arteriosus is suggested if the ratio exceeded 1.28 +/-.23 compared with normal premature values of 0.87 +/-.12.

Indirect M-Mode estimates of cardiac function

Fractional Shortening: Although formulas are available for calculation of Pediatric LV volumes [Volume = -19.1 + 14.6 x Be + .062 x Be^3 (Be= LV lateral minor axis on echo;^ = raised to the power of)], accurate estimates of LV contractility may be obtained by calculation of Fractional Shortening (FS) where:

FS=(LVED Dimension-LVES Dimension)/LVED Dimension
[LVED=LV end diastolic/ LVES=LV end systolic]

Henry's data reflect a normal range of 28-44% (average = 36%). One use of FS arises in a group of premature infants with PDA where the presence of PDA without heart failure was associated with increased FS, which returned to normal upon closure of the PDA. In the group with congestive heart failure, FS was normal or decreased. Serial measurements are required in any one patient.

Mean Vcf: This measurement is:

Fractional Shortening /Ejection Time (secs)

It is expressed in circumferences/sec. LV ejection time in children is ordinarily easily determined as the interval between aortic valve opening and closing. LV posterior wall motion or mitral valve closure are other less accurate methods to determine ejection time. Sahn reported a range of mean Vcf in newborns of 0.92-2.2 circ/sec with an average of 1.51 +/-.04 circ/sec. Other interesting associations for Vcf are:

1.34 +/-.03 : Children 5-15 years old
2.12 +/-.08 : Children with large Left to Right Shunts
1.18 +/-.06 : Infants with Congestive Heart Failure

Mitral regurgitation or dyskinetic LV wall motion renders Vcf an inaccurate estimate of function. It is generally not useful to determine the severity of aortic stenosis.

Systolic Time Intervals: Determination of Left or Right Ventricular Systolic Time Intervals (LVSTI or RVSTI) requires adequate visualization of both aortic and pulmonary valves, accurate recording of M-Mode tracings at a paper speed of 75-100 mm/sec and time lines usually at less than 100 msec intervals.

A Ventricle's Systolic Time Interval (sec) is:

Pre-Ejection Period (PEP)/ Ejection Time (ET)

PEP is the interval between the initial portion of the QRS deflection on an ECG and cusp opening of the semi-lunar valve. ET is the interval between cusp opening and closing.

LVPEP/LVET= .35 (range .30-.39) sec
RVPEP/RVET= .24 (range .16-.30) sec

Generally, as afterload increases, PEP increases and ET decreases. An increases in RVPEP/RVET reflects an increase in pulmonary arterial diastolic pressure, whereby a ratio of greater than 0.3 usually reflects a diastolic pulmonary arterial pressure of greater than 30 mm Hg. Useful extensions of the above relationships include the non-invasive evaluation of pulmonary vascular reactivity in patients with increased pulmonary vascular resistance. In patients with reactive increases in pulmonary vascular resistance one would expect a decreased RVPEP/RVET upon administration of oxygen, compared with room air values.

Isovolumic Contraction Time (IVT): This measurement represents the interval between mitral valve closure to aortic cusp opening. One study correlated this interval with age and heart rate as follows:

22 +/- 9 msec: Children < 3 Years
33 +/- 7 msec: Children > 3 Years
19 +/- 5 msec: Heart Rates >130 Beats/min
33 +/- 6 msec: Heart Rates 70-130 Beats/min

Patients with LV myocardial disease had increased IVT as follows:

49 +/- 12 msec: Age <3 Years and HR >130
62 +/- 21 msec: Age >3 Years and HR 70-130

In patients with PDA, the IVT decreased to 12 +/- 4 msec in children less than 3 years and to 17 +/- 9 msec in children older than 3 years.

LV posterior wall motion velocity or percent shortening of the LV free wall have not been studied in detail in infants and children. For further reading, many excellent pediatric M-mode echocardiography texts are available (5,6,7).

Real Time or Cross-Sectional Echocardiographic Imaging

It is this form of imaging that has enabled elegant elaboration of intracardiac anatomy. Diagnostic information relating to lesions such as hypoplastic left heart syndrome, tetralogy of Fallot, complete transposition of the great vessels, tricuspid atresia, Ebstein anomaly, complete atrioventricular canal defects, aortic coarctation, atrial septal defect, ventricular septal defect, and patent ductus arteriosus is excellent. In many centers, surgical correction of lesions such as aortic coarctation and complete atrioventricular canal defects is possible without diagnostic cardiac catheterization. In the instance of complete atrioventricular canal defects, this approach assumes that the child is young enough [i.e., less than six to nine months of age] so that the physician knows that irreversible pulmonary vascular disease is not present. It is also interesting to note that real-time imaging provides more useful information about the exact structure of the atrioventricular valves than does angiocardiography.

MAGNETIC RESONANCE IMAGING [MRI]

This new exciting imaging tool supplements information we are now accustomed to obtaining on real time echocardiography. Specifically, it appears to provide excellent details of the entire aortic arch, allowing elaboration of vascular rings, aortic dilatation such as occurs in patients with Marfan Syndrome, anomalous subclavian arteries [this is critical information prior to surgical palliation of tetralogy of Fallot, when it becomes important to avoid the anomalous subclavian for aortico-pulmonary anastomosis], and anomalous pulmonary venous return. These are structures imaged by real time echocardiography, but often incompletely. Post-operative evaluation of repairs for complete transposition and other lesions is another potential use. Importantly, although areas of anatomical narrowing image with this technique, information relating to the exact degree of obstruction is not provided. Newer Doppler techniques, however, can provide this physiological information. An important limitation of this technology is that the presence of any large metallic object is not possible, so that a patient requiring mechanical ventilation would not be a candidate for this imaging with present systems. It is possible that temporary plastic support devices may even allow study of ventilator dependent patients.

DOPPLER ECHOCARDIOGRAPHY

Whereas the selective combination of cross-sectional or real-time echocardiography with magnetic resonance imaging elaborates the vast majority of significant intracardiac and great vessel anatomy, the addition to these imaging capabilities of Doppler flow analysis allows estimation of physiological data as well. Validation of the accuracy of maximum instantaneous pressure differences across the aortic and pulmonary valves is established. Estimates of subaortic tunnel stenosis is less accurate because of limitations of the technique in long segment narrowing. Detection of atrioventricular valve insufficiency with semi-quantification, detection of ventricular septal defect flow, detection of patent ductus arteriosus flow, are all possible. Atrial septal defect flow is also possible but less exact.

One must be aware of the fact that instantaneous maximum pressure difference across a semilunar valve differs from the maximum peak to peak systolic pressure difference across the valve as measured during cardiac catheterization. The latter value had been the absolute standard used to make decisions for operative intervention relating to aortic or pulmonary valve stenosis. The author predicts that once data from Doppler examination are standardized and further correlated with previous cardiac catheterization data, Doppler assessment of the severity of aortic or pulmonary stenosis will likely replace diagnostic cardiac catheterization.

It is also interesting that one is able to demonstrate minimal tricuspid regurgitation in the majority of patients studied, although no clinical tricuspid insufficiency is present. This likely represents the spectrum of normal variation. Similarly in early studies with Doppler, pulmonary insufficiency was suspected in many normal persons. There is now some information suggesting that this finding represents coronary arterial flow in proximity with the pulmonary valve, in many normal subjects, and not true pulmonary insufficiency.

CARDIAC RADIOGRAPHS

With newer technologies including ECHO-DOPPLER studies, the true indications for cardiac radiographs are very limited. Most often, one derives the necessary information to supplement other studies and clinical findings with only a PA and lateral radiograph of the chest, whereas prior to ECHO, one most often ordered a cardiac series which included left and right anterior oblique projections, with inclusion of a barium filled esophagus. If one considers a vascular ring, a cardiac series is still desirable. Major areas of information relating to the utility of chest radiographs include the following:

[1] Evaluation of cardiomegaly: One common error is for a physician to order AP/lateral chest radiographs in the newborn with a suspicious cardiac murmur. Most often murmurs in the newborn are benign and even if not, radiographic determination of cardiomegaly is limited by large thymic shadows in this age. Exceptions include infants with complete transposition of the great vessels who are known to have little thymic tissue even at birth, likely because of stress. Furthermore, chest radiographs at any age should be obtained in an upright position to more accurately evaluate true cardiomegaly. This is even possible in the newborn using Plexiglas apparatus to stabilize an upright position. Studies performed in recumbent, restrained positions have little utility in the author's opinion. Generally, ECHO studies adequately demonstrate increased chamber dimension and therefore, cardiomegaly.

[2] Assessment of individual cardiac chamber enlargement: Evidence for right atrial enlargement occurs with prominence of the right inferior cardiac margin on PA projection. Left atrial enlargement often results in a double density within the right atrial shadow as well as upturning of the left mainstem bronchus. Right ventricular enlargement is best noted on the lateral projection and results in anterior impingement on the sternum by the anterior right ventricle to at least one half the length of the sternum, whereas the right ventricle ordinarily impinges only about one-third the distance between the inferior sternum and the superior sternum. Further evidence of right ventricular enlargement is upturning of the cardiac apex on PA projection. This is quite typical for tetralogy of Fallot. Once again, individual chamber enlargement is much more precisely determined using ECHO dimensions, which include wall and septal thicknesses.

These last two dimensions are obviously not possible using plain radiographic techniques. Left ventricular or left atrial enlargement manifests protrusion of the posterior cardiac shadow very posteriorly on left anterior oblique projections. Left ventricular enlargement often results in a squared off contour of the left lateral cardiac shape.

[3] Evaluation of pulmonary vascular markings: Increases or decreases in pulmonary vascular markings are a very useful determination of all the possible determinations on radiographic studies. Basic left to right shunts associated with increased pulmonary arterial pressures result in increased vascular markings. Interestingly, high pulmonary blood flow associated with normal pressures such as in patients with atrial septal defect, may often have normal pulmonary vascular markings early in childhood. Patients with complete transposition and tricuspid atresia with no associated pulmonary stenosis, uniformly have increased pulmonary vascular markings. Patients with tetralogy of Fallot and other complex lesions associated with severe pulmonary stenosis have oligemic lung fields, i.e., decreased pulmonary vascular markings. Although echocardiography allows determination of the proximal pulmonary arterial calibers, it is only indirectly possible to assess pulmonary blood flow by using additional Doppler technique. It is actually somewhat easier to determine whether a given patient has increase or decreased pulmonary blood flow by radiographic technique.

[4] Assessment of possible congestive cardiac failure: The classical triad in the suspicion of congestive heart failure [CHF] includes tachycardia, tachypnea, and cardiomegaly. One exception to the finding of cardiomegaly with overt CHF is obstructed total anomalous pulmonary venous return below the diaphragm. However almost all other lesions associated with CHF will manifest cardiomegaly. One must also assess central venous engorgement and congestive changes symmetrically pointing toward the hilum. It is occasionally impossible to completely distinguish CHF from certain forms of pneumonia and from increased pulmonary blood flow not associated with overt CHF. Clinical evaluation usually allows this distinction, however.

[5] Noting typical cardiac contours associated with classical malformation: The classical example of possible exact radiographic diagnosis is tetralogy of Fallot, where one notes an upturned cardiac apex secondary to RV enlargement, a decreased pulmonary artery segment from

small pulmonary arteries associated with severe pulmonary stenosis, and decreased pulmonary vascular markings. In 25% of patients with tetralogy of Fallot [and in truncus arteriosus] one additionally notes a right aortic arch. The overall configuration of the cardiac silhouette in these patients appears like a boot, hence the term "coeur en sabot." Patients with tricuspid atresia often have cardiac silhouettes that resemble an apple on a stick. Patients with complete transposition often have a very narrow mediastinum because the usual pulmonary arterial segment of the left lateral cardiac border is missing. In patients beyond 3-5 years of age with aortic coarctation, one often notes rib notching along the anterior first one-third of the ribs, secondary to collateral flow along the internal mammary arteries. Barium esophagrams in these patients often demonstrates an "E" sign, representing pre- and post-stenotic dilatation of the descending aorta. Ascending aortic prominence is present in patients with aortic stenosis and/or aortic insufficiency. Most other congenital defects manifest non-specific findings on radiographic exam, whereas echocardiographic exam is definitive in most instances.

In summary, radiographic examination of the pediatric cardiac patient is seldom necessary for accurate diagnosis but may contribute to an understanding of the physiological status in instances of increased or decreased pulmonary blood flow and in instances of congestive cardiac failure. The author no longer orders routine chest radiographs on any pediatric cardiology patient, and rarely finds radiographic study necessary other than the few instances noted in the discussion above. The disadvantage of this approach is missing non-cardiac chest pathology such as bronchogenic cysts or tumor. However, these are fortunately rare and do not present with primary cardiac concerns or findings.

Notes

1. Balady, GJ: How Physical Conditioning Affects the Electrocardiograms of Professional Football Players. *Primary Cardiology* p 122, December, 1985.

2. Henry WL, Gardin JM, Ware JH: Echocardiographic Measurements in Normal Subjects from Infancy to Old Age. *Circulation* 62: 1054, 1980.

3. Haycock GB, Schwartz GJ, Wisotsky DH: Geometric method for measuring body surface area: A height-weight formula validated in infants, children, and adults. *J Peds* 93:62, 1978.

4. Sahn DJ, DeMario A, Kisslo J, Weyman A: The Committee on M-Mode Standardization of the American Society of Echocardiography. Recommendations Regarding Quantitation in M-Mode Echocardiography: Results of a Survey of Echocardiographic Measurements. *Circulation* 58:1072, 1978.

5. Goldberg JG, Allen HD, Sahn DJ: *Pediatric and Adolescent Echocardiography*: A Handbook. Chicago, Year Book Medical Publishers, Inc., 1975.

6. Meyer, RA: *Pediatric Echocardiography.* Philadelphia, Lea & Febiger, 1977.

7. Williams RG, Tucker CR: *Echocardiographic Diagnosis of Congenital Heart Disease*. Boston, Little, Brown and Company, 1977.

Chapter 4

Invasive Tools

The classical invasive tool pertaining to pediatric cardiology remains *cardiac catheterization*. However, with the advent of excellent non-invasive imaging techniques and accurate physiological determinations such as instantaneous pressure differences across stenotic semi-lunar valves by Doppler, the indications for this procedure have changed. Pre-operative anatomical definition remains important, although many surgeons are willing to perform total operative repair of such lesions as uncomplicated complete atrioventricular canal [A-V Canal], atrial septal defect [ASD], patent ductus arteriosus [PDA], and Aortic Coarctation provided there is no evidence of a more complex associated lesion. Physiological assessment of pulmonary vascular resistance remains important in the older patient with pulmonary hypertension from any cause such as ventricular septal defect or patent ductus arteriosus. Interventional cardiac cath procedures such as balloon dilation of pulmonary stenosis or of aortic stenosis are beginning to replace the simple diagnostic cardiac catheterizations. Balloon atrial septostomy in the newborn with complete transposition of the great vessels was the earliest interventional cath procedure and is still performed. Blade atrial septostomies are now possible as well.

Basic Cardiac Cath Data: Before any logical discussion of cardiac cath data is possible, several concepts relating to oxygen in blood must be defined. The easiest way to understand the *total oxygen content* in blood is to equate it with the inorganic chemistry concept of *concentration*. In the instance of oxygen content the concentration of the substance of interest is a gas, not a solid. Therefore total oxygen content in a sample of blood is expressed in ml/liter in lieu of mg/liter. Adult cardiologists often measure content in volumes% or ml of oxygen/100 cc of blood. The total oxygen content in a sample of blood consists of two components:

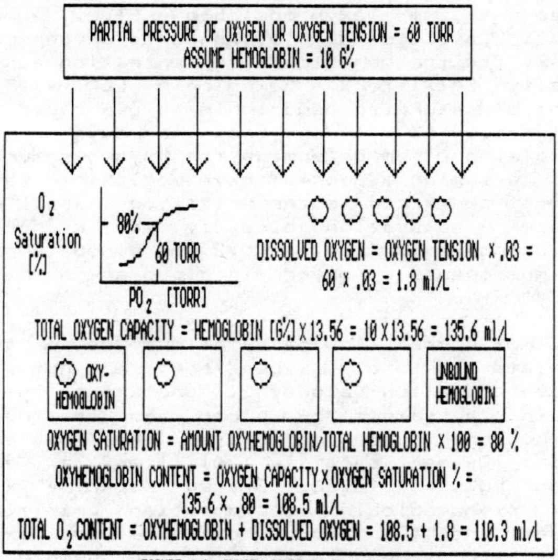

FIGURE 4.1: OXYGEN CONTENTS IN WHOLE BLOOD

[1] *oxyhemoglobin* [ml/L] or that portion of oxygen in a blood sample directly bound to hemoglobin and

[2] *dissolved* oxygen [ml/L] which relates directly to the partial pressure of oxygen in a sample of blood, reported as pO_2 in units of Torr or mm Hg. For every 100 Torr [or mm Hg] partial pressure of oxygen in a sample of blood, 3 ml/liter of oxygen is dissolved in the sample of blood. Therefore, .03 x oxygen tension [Torr] = the amount of dissolved oxygen in a sample of blood [ml/L]. The total possible amount of oxyhemoglobin [i.e., at 100% saturation], in a blood sample, known as oxygen capacity, relates solely to the hemoglobin concentration as follows: oxygen capacity [ml/liter] = hemoglobin [g%] x 13.56. The actual amount of saturated hemoglobin/oxygen capacity x 100 = oxygen saturation [%]. If one knows the oxygen tension in a blood sample, one can determine the oxygen saturation in that sample, assuming a normal oxyhemoglobin dissociation curve. In most pediatric catheterization labs, one can measure oxygen saturation directly by micro-oximeter techniques, using as little as 0.2 ml blood. Concepts of the various components of oxygen in blood are summarized in Figure 4.1.

All concepts of blood flow calculations using the Fick principle relate to total oxygen content, not to oxyhemoglobin concentration alone. If one knows the *oxygen saturation* in a sample of blood and the hemoglobin concentration, one can calculate the oxyhemoglobin concentration. Oxygen capacity [ml/liter] = Hemoglobin concentration [g%] x 13.56. Oxygen capacity x *oxygen saturation* = oxyhemoglobin concentration [ml/liter]. To this one must add the amount of dissolved oxygen as determined by the oxygen tension in the sample [oxygen tension (Torr) x .03 = dissolved oxygen(ml/L)]. In most cases, with the patient breathing room air, there will be very small differences between the amount of arterial and venous dissolved oxygen. For this reason, one can usually ignore dissolved oxygen in the calculation of arterial and venous oxygen content differences, and estimate total content by using only the oxyhemoglobin concentration. However, *one cannot ignore dissolved oxygen if the patient breathes a high concentration of oxygen during the catheterization* as is often the case when assessing pulmonary vascular reactivity.

The easiest way to think of blood flow calculations using the Fick principle is to remember the inorganic chemistry equation:

Amount [mg] = Concentration [mg/liter]/ Volume [liter]. Solving for volume [V]: V = Amount/Concentration. Taking the first derivative of both sides with respect to time, one derives:

[The change in Volume]/time = [Amount/time]/ [The change in Concentration]. Substituting a gas measurement [ml] for a solid measurement [mg], one finally has:

[The change in Volume]/time [liters/min] = Amount of oxygen consumed per minute [i.e., VO_2 or oxygen consumption]/ [Arterial-Venous Oxygen Content Differences [ml/liter]]. [The change in volume] = Flow [L/min]. It is this equation that has been the source of all blood flow calculations [Fig. 4.2]. Simply stated, if one knows the concentration differences across a given circulation and the amount of indicator lost or consumed [oxygen consumption], one can calculate the flow. One assumes that oxygen consumption equals the amount of oxygen delivered, and from this assumption, one can derive equations for calculations of pulmonary [Qp] and systemic [Qs] blood flows, including pure left to right [L-R] and right to left [R-L] shunts. To consider bidirectional shunting one needs to invoke a concept known as Effective Pulmonary Blood Flow [Qep]. The following definitions are useful in understanding notions of shunting and concepts of effective pulmonary blood flow:

[1] Pulmonary Blood Flow [Qp=L/min]: The total amount of blood entering the pulmonary circulation [pulmonary artery] and returning to the pulmonary veins.

[2] Systemic Blood Flow [Qs=L/min]: The total amount of blood flow entering the systemic circulation [aorta] and returning to the systemic great veins [Inferior and Superior Vena Cavae].

[3] Effective Pulmonary Blood Flow [Qep=L/min]: The amount of blood flow with systemic mixed venous oxygen saturation [and content] that enters the pulmonary circulation or the amount of blood flow with pulmonary venous oxygen saturation [and content] that enters the systemic circulation. This very important calculation allows determination of bidirectional [left to right and right to left] shunts when present. In the instance of isolated left to right shunt, the Qep equals the Qs; in the instance of isolated right to left shunt, the Qep equals the Qp.

[4] Left to Right Shunt [Q_{L-R}=L/min]: The amount of blood flow with pulmonary venous oxygen saturation [and content] that re-enters the pulmonary circulation.

[5] Right to Left Shunt [Q_{R-L}=L/min]: The amount of blood flow with systemic mixed venous oxygen saturation [and content] that re-enters the systemic circulation.

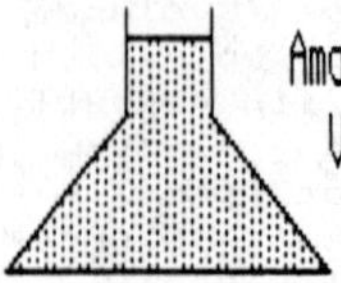

Amount[mg]=Concentration[mg/L] × Volume[L]

Volume[L]=Amount[mg]/ Concentration[mg/L]

With oxygen, amount would be expressed as ml instead of mg and concentration would be expressed in ml/L instead of mg/L

Flow=Volume/time [min]

Oxygen consumption [$\dot{V}O_2$] is the <u>amount</u> of oxygen consumed and delivered over time [min]

Note derivation of final Fick Equation indexed for surface area [square meters]:

$$\text{Flow [L/min/M}^2\text{]} = \dot{V}O_2\text{[ml/min/M}^2\text{]} \;/\; \text{[Arterial-Venous Contents]}_{\text{[ml/L]}}$$

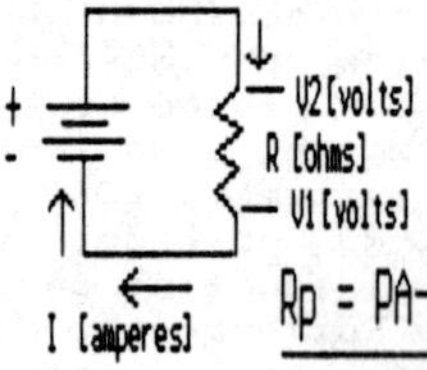

$$I = V2-V1 \;/\; R \text{ or } R = V2-V1 \;/\; I$$

Note that current is a flow of electrons and that voltage is analogous to pressure in a circulation.

Note similarity of pulmonary vascular resistance [units/M2] equation:

$$\text{Rp} = \text{PA-LA mean pressures/ Pulmonary Blood Flow per M}^2$$

FIG 4.2:FICK EQUATION AND RESISTANCE CONCEPTS

With further thought, one concludes that a left to right shunt increases the usual oxygen saturation and content between any point along proximal systemic venous return and the pulmonary arteries, and that an intracardiac [as opposed to an intrapulmonary] right to left shunt decreases the usual oxygen saturation and content between any point in the pulmonary venous return and the systemic arteries. Using these concepts during cardiac catheterization, one estimates an intracardiac left to right shunt based upon the detection of an increase in oxygen saturation and content during an oxygen saturation series [sampling series] from the superior and inferior vena cavae to the right and left pulmonary arteries; similarly a right to left shunt would manifest a decrease in oxygen saturation [compared with pulmonary venous oxygen saturation] at any point in the systemic circulation.

Nearly every pediatric cardiac cath procedure will include a complete right and left sided oxygen saturation series with calculation of pulmonary, systemic, effective pulmonary, left to right, and right to left blood flows. Other methods to detect intracardiac shunting include indicator dilution techniques such as thermodilution curves or actual angiocardiography with contrast material.

In addition to sampling oxygen saturation and/or blood gases or oxygen contents at various sites, the pediatric cardiologist measures pressure at important sites as well. These usually include superior vena cava, right atrium, right ventricle, main pulmonary artery, right and left pulmonary arteries, pulmonary arterial wedge pressures [catheter wedged at the most distal portion of the pulmonary artery in order to estimate left atrial pressures], left ventricle, ascending and descending aorta [Table 4.1].

Table 4.1: Normal Pediatric Cardiac Chamber and Vessel Pressures [mm Hg] (1)

CHAMBER	NEONATAL	POST-NEONATAL
Right Atrium	mean 0-4	a 5-8; v 2-6 mean 2-6
Right Ventricle	35-80/1-5	15-25/2-5
Pulmonary Artery	35-80/20-50 mean 25-60	15-25/8-12 mean 10-16
Pulmonary Wedge	-----	a 6-12; v 8-15 mean 5-12
Left Atrium	----- mean 3-6	a 6-12, v8-15 mean 5-10
Left Ventricle	-----	80-130/5-10
Systemic Artery	65-80/45-60 mean 60-65	90-130/60-80 mean 70-95

It is possible to measure direct left atrial pressures in the 25% of patients with a probe patent foramen ovale. Those patients with increased left atrial return from lesions such as PDA or VSD or with left ventricular obstructive lesions such as severe aortic stenosis or aortic coarctation seldom have a probe patent foramen ovale. Obviously the left atrium also could be entered in cases of atrial septal defect.

Using blood flow and pressure data, one is able to calculate vascular resistances. Whereas one could derive blood flow equations from inorganic chemistry concepts, one can derive equations for vascular resistance from direct current [DC] electrical circuit equations [Fig. 4.2].

Remember: I [electron flow or current in amperes] = V [voltage in volts]/ R [resistance in ohms], i.e., I = V/R. Solving for resistance one derives: R = V/I.

The physiological equations for vascular resistance are: R [Wood Units/m^2]= Mean Pressure Differences [mm Hg]/ Blood Flow [L/min/m^2]. For pulmonary vascular resistance [Rp]: Rp = [Mean pulmonary arterial pressure - mean left atrial pressure] / Pulmonary blood flow [Qp]. For systemic vascular resistance [Rs]: Rs = [Mean systemic arterial pressure - mean right atrial pressure] / Systemic blood flow [Qs]. The important calculation of pulmonary vascular resistance often involves decisions as to safety of operability in children with pulmonary hypertension of long duration, from any cause. Generally, if pulmonary vascular/systemic vascular resistance ratio exceeds .5 to .6, one could conclude that irreversible pulmonary vascular disease exists and operative intervention is not possible apart from consideration of future heart and lung transplants. If resting pulmonary vascular resistance is greater than 3-4 units/m^2, then repeat measurements of pulmonary blood flow as well as pulmonary arterial and wedge pressures are necessary during administration of tolazoline [into pulmonary arteries] and oxygen [by efficient mask] to assess whether these pulmonary vasodilators cause an increase in pulmonary blood flow and therefore a decrease in pulmonary vascular resistance into an operable range. These indications for cardiac cath have decreased markedly as advances in surgical capabilities allow earlier correction of complex congenital defects of the heart. Irreversible pulmonary vascular disease does not occur at sea level earlier than 18 months of age, usually. It could occur earlier at altitudes such as exist in Denver and Mexico City, and in infants with Down Syndrome, it occasionally occurs as early as six months of age. Early occurrence is also a problem in children with complete transposition of the great vessels, where irreversible pulmonary vascular disease has been reported in infants less than one year of age.

The final aspect of conventional pediatric cardiac catheterizations involves imaging. Ordinarily, biplane cineangiographic imaging, with C arm capabilities, allows definition of all complex congenital defects of the heart.

Interestingly, real-time echocardiography provides more exact anatomical relationships and definition of the atrio-ventricular valves attachments, compared with radiographic imaging.

Pre-catheterization [cath] orders: Before cardiac cath, the following are usually obtained, depending upon the cardiologists preference: Complete blood count to include indexes, urinalysis, BUN, creatinine, serum electrolytes [with particular attention to potassium if the patients is taking digitalis], recent ECG, recent echocardiogram; radiographs of the chest are optional and seldom obtained by the author because radiographic imaging of the heart and great vessels at the time of cath usually serves the same purpose as plain films of the thorax. If the patient is very polycythemic [hematocrit >55%], maintenance intravenous fluids are started using 5% glucose in 0.2 normal saline solution, once the patient is not taking anything further by mouth [usually 2 a.m. if cardiac cath is scheduled as first case the following morning; otherwise at least six to eight hours before the procedure]. Digitalis is held the evening before cardiac cath in order to minimize arrhythmias during the procedure. Some centers do not follow this precaution. Diuretic therapy is also stopped on the evening prior to the cath to avoid dehydration in face of the use of contrast material for angiographic procedures. Obviously informed consent must be obtained prior to such a procedure, which generally has a low risk of catastrophic complications. In the infant with little or no cyanosis, pre-cath sedation usually involves combinations of Demerol [meperidine, 2 mg/kg], Phenergan [promethazine, 1mg/Kg], and Thorazine [chlorpromazine, 1 mg/kg]. This sedation is quite strong and one might consider Demerol [1-2 mg/kg] with Vistaril [1 mg/kg] alone. All medications may be given intramuscularly. In the cyanotic patient, especially with the potential for a hypercyanotic spell, one may consider morphine sulfate 0.1-0.2 mg/kg IM or subcutaneously. Children less than six months of age generally receive no sedation or small doses of morphine alone. Some centers resort to general anesthesia for cath procedures. The author opposes this approach because of the marked effects general anesthesia has upon hemodynamics and myocardial performance, and because of the inherent risks of general anesthesia.

Post cath orders: After cardiac cath one monitors vital signs closely for one to three hours, usually every fifteen minutes. If stable, vital signs may be obtained every two to four hours, thereafter. Monitoring of peripheral pulses in the extremity involved in arterial entry, is essential, and the nurse should communicate any significant decrease to the cardiologist or resident. If one ordered light sedation, then a regular diet could be resumed after establishing that the child tolerates clear liquids. One may resume pre-cath medications as well. If there are no apparent arterial or rhythm problems, we discharge children during late afternoon or early evening on the day of a morning procedure if no further intervention is anticipated, provided the cath itself was not interventional [e.g., relief of pulmonary stenosis by balloon dilatation], and provided one notes normal urination if the child received contrast material.

Complications: Complications after cardiac cath usually involve ooze or bleeding from the cath site, transient decrease in the peripheral pulses of the extremity of arterial entry, and/or transient temperature increase from mild dehydration and the osmotic effects of contrast material [newer low osmotic agents are becoming available]. Because the procedure is sterile, bacterial endocarditis is not a major risk, unless contamination develops. In this event, SBE prophylaxis is necessary, whereas this is not usually the case.

During the procedure, one may observe significant arrhythmias, including complete heart block [especially in children with corrected transposition or truncus arteriosus], severe bradycardia, supraventricular tachycardia, ventricular tachycardia and ventricular fibrillation. Perforation of a chamber is possible if manipulation of a stiff catheter is vigorous. Atrial appendages and right ventricular outflow regions are particularly vulnerable to perforation. In such instances the catheter should be left in place and removed under surgical control. Knotting of a catheter is possible. Allergic reaction to contrast material may be as severe as penicillin anaphylactic reactions. Death in association with cath is rare, especially in children older than six months of age, and generally occurs in 1 out of 10,000 studies.

Interventional Cardiac Catheterization: Interventional procedures now include balloon dilatation relief of pulmonary valve stenosis [excluding dysplastic valves], balloon dilatation relief of aortic stenosis in selected instances [we still fear the degree of aortic insufficiency that may result], blade atrial septostomy, balloon atrial septostomy, and balloon dilatation relief of aortic coarctation. Balloon dilatation of aortic coarctation, whether primary of for recoarctation after surgery, should not be performed until more data is available regarding safety of this particular procedure. There are now reports of late aneurysm formation in the region of original coarctation, three to five years after original procedure. Surgical relief of such aneurysms then becomes complicated by the fact that relief of the coarctation by balloon dilatation results in regression of collateral vessel flow. There have also been several deaths and cerebrovascular accidents in association with this procedure. Surgical repair of aortic coarctation has become very safe in comparison.

Also included in interventional procedures are endomyocardial muscle biopsies to aid in the diagnosis and management of cardiomyopathies, and to evaluate the myocardial state after cardiac transplantation. Non-surgical closure of atrial septal defect and of patent ductus arteriosus have been possible, but the author considers these approaches less desirable than surgical intervention at this time, because of complications and incomplete closure of these defects. Occlusion of pulmonary arterio-venous malformations as exist in Rendu-Osler-Weber syndrome [familial hemorrhagic telangiectasia], is possible by use of latex balloons, in lieu of surgical resection. Removal of right atrial or right ventricular foreign bodies is usually possible by catheter techniques, in order to avoid surgical removal.

Electrophysiological studies [EPS]: Although more experience exists in the adult population, most large pediatric cardiology services include an electrophysiologist, who is capable of performing sophisticated EPS studies. Such studies aid in exact therapeutic choices for complex cardiac arrhythmias such as automatic atrial tachycardia, aid in the exact diagnoses of complex arrhythmias, and importantly may include electrical ablation of arrhythmogenic foci. Complications are similar to those listed under cardiac catheterization.

Notes

1. Rudolph AM [ed], Hoffman JIE [coed]: *Pediatrics*, 7th Edition. Norwalk, Appleton-Century-Crofts, 1982, p 1260.

Chapter 5

Perinatal Aspects of Pediatric Cardiology

Fetal Circulation: One can best consider the fetal circulation by understanding that the fetal lung, which is airless and essentially collapsed in utero, is replaced by the umbilical-placental circulation. Flows with the average lowest oxygen contents are delivered to the placenta by the umbilical arteries [two in most instances] from the descending aorta, and flows with the average highest oxygen content are returned to the inferior vena cava after portions variably divide into ductus venosus and intrahepatic circulations. Because of anatomical angulation of the inferior vena cava toward the left atrium, inferior vena cava flow is directed in large part to the left atrium, across the freely patent foramen ovale. Therefore, flow with the relatively highest intracardiac oxygen content reaches the left atrium and left ventricle for ejection into the aorta, where the coronary arteries and brachiocephalic vessels receive this relatively saturated flow.

Almost the entire flow returning from the head and neck into the superior vena cava is diverted around the IVC flow within the right atrium to reach the right ventricle and pulmonary artery. Once in the pulmonary artery, the extremely high fetal pulmonary vascular resistance allows only about 6% of combined ventricular output to circulate into the pulmonary circulation, with the remainder flowing across a widely patent ductus arteriosus into the descending aorta where it may again reach the umbilical-placental circulation. Thus in general terms and after mixing occurs, the fetal circulation provides for flow with the most oxygen content to reach the coronary arteries and brachiocephalic vessels and for flow with the least oxygen content to reach the descending aorta and umbilical-placental circulation. The notion of fetal right ventricular dominance whereby the right ventricle ejects 55-65% of the combined fetal ventricular output compared with a left ventricular output of 35-45%, has been fascinatingly reconfirmed recently in the human fetus using Doppler techniques.

Although the above circulation appears desirable, it is important to realize that the overall differences between oxygen tensions and contents in the aorta and pulmonary artery of the fetus are not great [18-19 torr in the pulmonary artery compared with 23-25 torr in the ascending aorta] and that lesions as significant as complete transposition of the great vessels where the aorta and pulmonary artery arise from the opposite of the usual ventricle are tolerated well by the fetus.

The following is a summary of oxygen tensions in the fetal circulation [torr]: umbilical vein 30-35; inferior vena cava 26-28; superior vena cava 12-14; pulmonary artery 18-19; ascending aorta 23-25; descending aorta 20-22 (1).

Transitional Circulation: Upon delivery, the fetus has the task of changing the organ of oxygen delivery from the placenta to the lungs. With the first breath, the newborn's lungs expand and the pulmonary arterioles unfold with an associated very significant decrease in pulmonary vascular resistance. Importantly, the pulmonary vascular resistance is still very high and very reactive because of thickened pulmonary arterioles compared with the child older than 4 to 6 weeks of age and the adult. As one clamps the umbilical cord, the systemic vascular resistance increases significantly. The significant decrease in pulmonary vascular resistance allows an increased pulmonary blood flow with concomitant increases in left atrial pressures as pulmonary venous return increases. Left atrial pressures are also increased because of the sudden increase in LV afterload from clamping of the umbilical chord, and therefore removing the low resistance umbilical-placental circulation. This increase in left atrial pressure tends to close the foramen ovale. The anatomically normal ductus arteriosus closes functionally within 18 hours of age and then undergoes further permanent closure resulting in a ligamentum arteriosum. This change then completes the transition from fetal to newborn circulation.

Persistent fetal circulation: Not all neonates are able to accomplish a smooth transition postnatally, especially if delivery is traumatic or associated with prolonged hypoxia or meconium aspiration. As noted above, although the newborn pulmonary vascular resistance is very much lower than it had been in utero, it is still relatively increased and very reactive to stimuli such as hypoxia, hypercarbia, and acidemia, all of which tend to constrict the pulmonary arterioles with a resulting further increase in pulmonary vascular resistance. Added to this potential marked increase in pulmonary vascular resistance is the fact that the newborn myocardium is very dependent upon substrate such as calcium and glucose for normal function and further compromised in functional capabilities by decreased sympathetic drive and a relatively high ratio of ground substance to myocardial fibers. The net result of these limitations are an inability for the newborn to increase stroke volume as a means of increasing cardiac output. Rather, the newborn must increase heart rate to achieve any significant increase in cardiac output.

In the newborn suffering from decreased metabolic substrate with hypoglycemia and/or hypocalcemia myocardial function is further decreased. If one then adds an hypoxic insult such as meconium aspiration, the further increase in pulmonary vascular resistance may be too great for the right ventricle to handle comfortably and the newborn will make an effort to alleviate the problem by utilizing pathways present during fetal development, such as the foramen ovale or patent ductus arteriosus. Polycythemia further accentuates the problem by increasing blood viscocity and indirectly increasing vascular resistances further. The stage is set, therefore, in a setting of hypoglycemia, hypocalcemia, polycythemia, or hypoxic insult such as meconium aspiration.

If the newborn uses fetal pathways such as the foramen ovale and patent ductus arteriosus, desaturated flow would reach the new systemic circulation and result in variable degrees of cyanosis. If the dominant flow is at the foramen level, then the entire systemic circulation would be desaturated [i.e., right and left radial and umbilical arterial or femoral arterial arterial blood gases would reflect similar levels of desaturation]. If the dominant flow is at the ductus arteriosus level from the main pulmonary to the descending aorta, then the upper extremity arterial samples would show little desaturation, compared with a very desaturated umbilical or femoral arterial samples. Because the left subclavian artery originates in relatively close proximity with the ductus arteriosus, left radial arterial samples are less reliable than right radial arterial samples for assessing these situations.

The pattern of persistent fetal circulation may be so severe as to result in death of the newborn and requires vigorous therapy including ventilatory support to correct hypercarbia and actually result in hypocarbia in an attempt to decrease pulmonary vascular resistance. Metabolic derangement such as hypocalcemia or hypoglycemia must be corrected at once as well. If all intervention fails, including possible use of tolazoline [which decreases pulmonary vascular resistance but may also decrease systemic vascular resistance] and dopamine to improve compromised myocardial performance, then some centers are beginning to offer extracorporeal membrane oxygen techniques [ECMO] to sustain such infants. The technique must be considered experimental and involves cannulation of the jugular vein and ipsilateral carotid artery with subsequent placement of the cannulae into the right atrium and ascending aorta. Desaturated systemic venous return is drained to the membrane oxygenator and a highly saturated flow is returned into the ascending aorta at appropriate flow rates. The infant is then weaned from this support and, upon discontinuation, the carotid artery and the jugular veins are ligated. One must question the long term outcome when the infant was so hypoxic for a sustained period prior to use of this technique, and the long term effects of ligation of a major cerebral vessel. Nevertheless, the technique is preliminarily useful. Its utility may be short lived if one considers the extreme therapeutic potential for a prostaglandin derivative or calcium channel blocker in the future management of persistent pulmonary hypertension or persistent fetal circulation.

Prematurity and bronchopulmonary dysplasia: Prematurity presents two major cardiovascular problems: [1] patent ductus arteriosus and [2] possible bronchopulmonary dysplasia. Most tertiary intensive care nurseries or perinatal centers have capabilities of surgical PDA ligation in the preterm infant directly in the nursery, if intravenous indomethacin in not effective or if there is a contraindication to its use. Detection of PDA in the premature infant involves clinical exam coupled with echocardiography and Doppler study, especially if there is a history of carbon dioxide retention or failure to wean from the ventilator.

Bronchopulmonary dysplasia often requires constant diuretic therapy [e.g., aldactone 2.2 mg/kg/day divided into q 8 h doses and chlorothiazide 15 mg/kg/dose q 12 h] and is associated with fluid sensitivity. Recent studies indicate an increase in antidiuretic hormone as a possible cause of fluid imbalance (2). Occasionally ventricular dysfunction develops and digoxin therapy is needed. One may also note cardiac hypertrophy of unexplained etiology. Pulmonary vascular resistance may be markedly increased upon late follow up (3).

Notes

1. Rudolph AM. Fetal Circulation and Cardiovascular Adjustments After Birth. In Rudolph AM [ed], Hoffman JIE [coed]: *Pediatrics*, 7th Edition. Norwalk, Appleton-Century-Crofts, 1982, pp 1231-1235.

2. Rao M, Eid N, Herrod L, Parekh A, Steiner P: Antidiuretic Hormone Response in Children With Bronchopulmonary Dysplasia During Episodes of Acute Respiratory Distress. *Am J Dis Child* 140:825-828, 1986.

3. Berman W Jr, Katz R, Yabek SM, Dillon T, Fripp RR, Papile L: Long-term follow-up of bronchopulmonary dysplasia. *J Pediatr* 109:45-50, 1986.

Chapter 6

Congenital Cardiac Defects

The various congenital cardiac defects in this chapter are organized according to their basic physiological similarities in order to promote an understanding of basic cardiac physiology. General concepts of anatomy, patient history, natural history, and physical findings associated with the common defects will appear for each of the major lesions in a physiological group. Subheadings reflect physiological groups. Less common defects will appear under their appropriate group, but discussions will not include redundant similarities to the most common defects in the group. Rather, the author will present the unique features of the more rare defects.

Before actual discussion of the individual defects, definition of some basic but usually confusing terms is necessary. The concept of cardiac looping involves development of the heart from a straight cardiac tube followed by gentle curving rightward [dextro or D-loop] or leftward [levo or L-loop]. Note that during embyrogenesis, the primitive ventricle [PV in Fig. 6.1] basically becomes the left ventricle and the bulbus cordis [BC in Fig. 6.1] basically becomes the right ventricle. With further curving and with both ventricle assuming an inferior position, D-loop results in an anatomical right ventricle on the right and an anatomical left ventricle on the left. This would be the normal ventricular relationship. With L-looping, the anatomical right ventricle is on the left and the anatomical left ventricle is on the right, resulting in ventricular inversion. Because the left atrium fills this left sided anatomical right ventricle and the aorta arises from this ventricle, pulmonary venous return reaches the aorta properly, although it is the anatomical right ventricle ejecting into the aorta. On the right, the right atrium fills the right sided, anatomical left ventricle, which ejects systemic venous return into the pulmonary artery. Because physiological flows are normal with

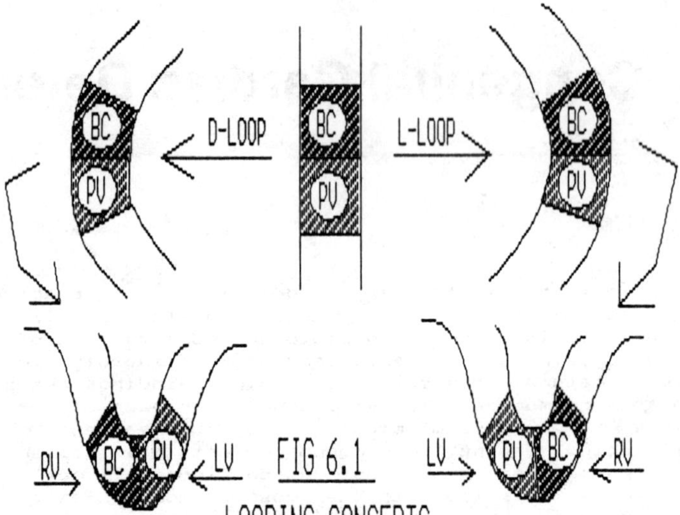

FIG 6.1

LOOPING CONCEPTS

pulmonary venous return entering the aorta and systemic venous return entering the pulmonary artery, this anatomical complex is known as "corrected transposition" or L-loop [ventricular inversion], L-transposition [aortic valve is anterior and to the left]. Interestingly, the ventricles bring with them the conduction system and atrio-ventricular valves developmentally so that with ventricular inversion septal depolarization occurs from right to left and results in possible q waves in leads V4R and V1, with no septal Q waves in leads V5-6. Furthermore the left sided atrio-ventricular valve is anatomically a tricuspid valve with the right sided atrio-ventricular valve being a mitral valve. Ebstein's malformation of the left sided, tricuspid valve is possible. If no other lesions are present such as VSD with or without pulmonary stenosis, patients with isolated "corrected transposition" may do quite well but are at significant risk of evolving complete heart block, progressing from first degree A-V block [refer to Chapter 3 on non-invasive tools under ECG discussion as well as figs. 6.1 and 6.2. The term transposition implies an anterior malposition of the aortic valve in relation to the pulmonary valve. In "complete transposition" or D-transposition, the aortic valve is anterior and to the right of the pulmonary valve and arises from a right sided, anatomical right ventricle [hence D-loop or normal ventricular relationship]. Following the course of blood in this instance one discovers that the right atrium drains systemic venous return to the right ventricle which ejects it into the aorta. The left atrium receives pulmonary venous return and carries it to the left ventricle which ejects it into the pulmonary artery. Obviously one has two separate parallel circulations requiring some point of admixture between the circulations for the patient to survive. See discussion on complete transposition below. Whatever semilunar valve arises from the right ventricle is anatomically superior in relationship to the other because of the outflow region in the right ventricle or infundibulum. This chamber was the *conus arteriosus* embryologically, and later separates from the right ventricular inflow chamber by the crista supraventricularis composed of the moderator, septal and parietal bands in the right ventricle. With no interposition of an infundibulum between the left ventricular chamber and the aortic valve, fibrous continuity of the mitral and aortic valves is possible. In the instance of double outlet right ventricle, the *conus arteriosus* divides nearly equally beneath both semilunar valves so that the aortic and pulmonary valve are at the same horizontal position in addition to being directly side by side on lateral projection [Fig. 6.2].

One other important notion involves the abdominal visceral relationships. Normally one has situs solitus with the liver on the right and the stomach on the left. Situs inversus indicates that the stomach is on the right and the liver is on the left. Some patients have an indeterminate situs with horizontal liver. This may occur in patients with asplenia and polysplenia syndromes. Most children with asplenia have transposition, severe pulmonary stenosis or atresia, atrioventricular septal defects or single ventricle, and two-thirds have anomalous pulmonary venous connection to vena cava or portal system. Such children are usually very cyanotic and are at risk of infection because of the absent spleen. There is right sided symmetry [absence of a left sided structure or spleen] with symmetrical right sided bronchial configuration or

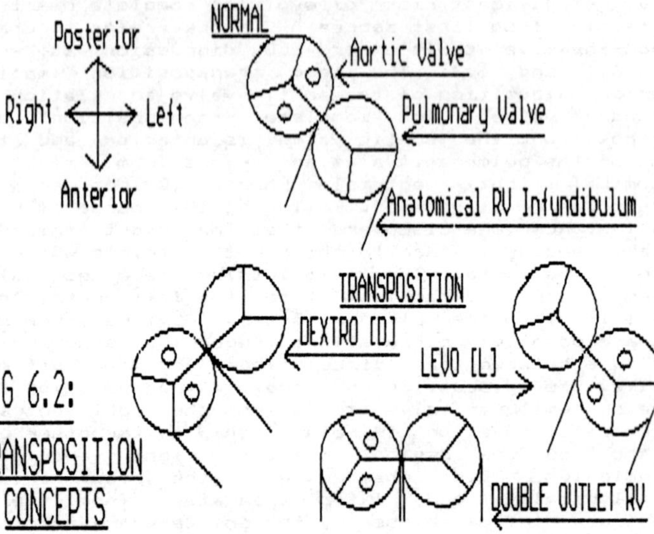

FIG 6.2: TRANSPOSITION CONCEPTS

bilateral middle lobes in the lungs. Children with polysplenia usually have large left to right shunts associated with atrial and ventricular septal defects, common atrioventricular septal defects with possible double outlet right ventricle. Aortic stenosis and coarctation are also possible but transposition or pulmonary stenosis are unusual. Pulmonary veins may connect to either or both atria and two-thirds have interrupted inferior vena cava with hemiazygous continuation (1). There is bilateral left sided symmetry [spleen is a left sided structure] including symmetrical left sided bronchial configuration and the possibility of two sinus nodes alternately discharging.

One last note involves interpretation of the representative physiology figures in this chapter. Representative intracardiac pressures are noted within rectangles whereas representative saturations are noted within circles. The less saturated a blood flow, the darker it appears, with flow from the lungs into the left atrium represented as white and fully saturated at 95-96%. Cyanotic lesions will have darker shaded flows into the aorta and common mixing lesions will have similar shaded flows entering the aorta and pulmonary artery, generally.

I. LEFT TO RIGHT SHUNTS AT THE ATRIAL LEVEL:

Atrial Septal Defect [Secundum]

Physiology: The most representative lesion in this group is the classical secundum atrial septal defect [ASD], or a defect in the atrial septum in the region of the foramen ovale. The physiological consequences of these defects relate largely to the magnitude of the left to right shunt at the atrial level [see definition and discussion of left to right shunts in Chapter 3 and Fig. 6.3]. The magnitude of left to right shunt at the atrial level depends largely upon relative left and right ventricular compliances. Although quite complex in theory, one could view compliance as a measure of how easy or difficult it is to fill a ventricle. A ventricle with high compliance would be easy to fill and one with a low compliance would be difficult to fill and by implication, more "stiff." Whereas ventricular compliance reflects ease of volume input, afterload reflects ease of volume ejection or output. Generally a ventricle facing a lower afterload, has a higher compliance. Therefore, the right ventricle facing the low pulmonary circulatory afterload ordinarily has a higher compliance [fills more easily] than the left ventricle facing the high systemic circulatory afterload. This differs in the immediate newborn period when the pulmonary vascular resistance is very high until a gradual decreased occurs over the first 6 to 8 postnatal weeks.

The above discussion of ventricular compliance should allow a more plausible explanation of the variability of the natural history of ASD. In the majority of children with usual large secundum ASD, manifestation of the defect is rare in infancy and early childhood. In fact, appreciation of the classical findings of ASD is usually not possible until the child is 2 to 4 years of age. This natural history reflects the fact that in the immediate newborn period, the magnitude of atrial left to right shunt

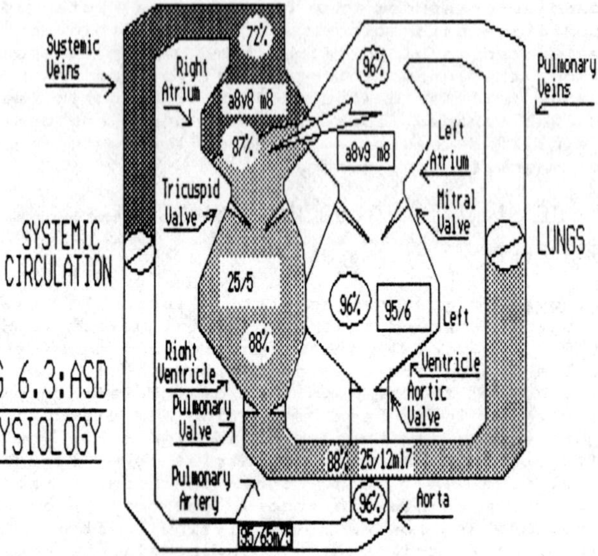

FIG 6.3:ASD PHYSIOLOGY

secondary to ASD is less compared with the child in whom the high neonatal pulmonary vascular resistance has decreased to normal. Even after this point, it is probable that it takes an even longer period for the ventricles to readjust their compliances as a reflection of the decreased pulmonary resistance. Furthermore the tendency of the right ventricle to become more compliant would be balanced by its tendency to hypertrophy in response to the volume load, which would result in a decreased compliance.

In a small group of infants, overt CHF develops in association with ASD. The explanation as to why this group differs likely involves an unusually large neonatal left to right shunt because of an unusually low left ventricular compliance or an unusually high right ventricular compliance. This large atrial shunt would be difficult for the neonatal cardiac muscle to handle because at this time, cardiac function is quite limited. The newborn has little ability to increase stroke volume, in part because of a higher proportion of ground substance to cardiac muscle at this age. Furthermore, cardiac sympathetic drive develops postnatally in the human and this would also compromise neonatal cardiac performance. It is also interesting to note that in this small group of ASD patients, spontaneous closure of the defect can occur, whereas this event is very unusual in the child that manifests ASD in the more usual later years.

Usual natural history: Apart from the small group that develops early CHF, the majority of children with ASD are asymptomatic regarding the C-V system. They theoretically should have a higher than usual incidence of pneumonias and upper respiratory infections; however, even this history is not usual. If missed during childhood, the patient with uncomplicated ASD often presents to a physician complaining of easy fatigue. The author believes that a low degree of easy fatigue also manifests in childhood, but it too subtle to recognize. This belief stems from the usual parental comment after repair of ASD in childhood that "We had no idea that our child could have so much energy, compared with his abilities before surgery." Because the left to right atrial shunt is low pressure and high volume, risk of irreversible pulmonary vascular disease is not present during childhood in most circumstances. This serious complication may occur any time after the second to third decade. It is not unusual, however, for a patient to reach the sixth or seventh decade and still have no significant pulmonary vascular damage.

Physical findings: The diagnosis of ASD can be quite difficult, even for the fully trained cardiologist. In childhood, the usual presentation is for evaluation of a cardiac murmur. On general exam, one might subtly note slight left precordial prominence. No compromise of growth is usually apparent, and the patient is not cyanotic. Vital signs and blood pressures are normal. On cardiac exam, one notes a significant RV heave at the lower left sternal border when the child is reclining. The apical impulse is normal and not hyperdynamic. The first heart sound is normal in the usual forms of ASD; the second heart sound is widely split and fixed during all phases of respiration with the child sitting. The pulmonary component is normal but occasionally appears louder than usual, likely because it is so separate from the aortic component and because the dilated pulmonary artery may transmit P2 more easily. A third sound is common along the left sternal border. The murmur is a slightly harsh, short pulmonary ejection murmur at the upper left sternal border, secondary to relative pulmonary stenosis in face of the very increased pulmonary blood flow. There is little radiation other than lateral radiation in early infancy associated with physiological peripheral pulmonary stenosis at that age. A mid diastolic rumble is present at the mid to lower left sternal border, reflecting relative tricuspid stenosis in face of the increased tricuspid flow. Because of a high incidence of associated mitral valve prolapse, an early or mid systolic click is often present between the apex and lower left sternal border.

The major differential diagnosis involves mild to moderate valvar pulmonic stenosis. In that group of patients, one is unable to appreciate a mid-diastolic rumble, the quality of the ejection murmur is usually more harsh, and there is an intermittent systolic ejection click over the pulmonary area at the upper left sternal border.

Pulses are usually normal and symmetrical. Although several texts mention a slight decrease in peripheral pulses in patients with ASD, the author has not consistently appreciated this finding.

<u>ECG findings</u>: Right axis deviation is usual. First degree A-V block is somewhat common [about 10% of patients] in secundum ASD, and is quite common in the ostium primum variant. QRS duration is normal. QTc interval is normal. The most typical finding is an rsR′ configuration in the right precordial leads V1/V4R, with associated slight prominence of rightward forces in the left precordial leads [S waves in leads V5/V6].

<u>Echo findings</u>: It is common to directly image a secundum atrial septal defect on cross-sectional echo. M-Mode findings include paradoxical septal motion [anterior systolic motion] and increased RV dimensions. The pulmonary arteries are prominent on real-time scan as well. If present, mitral valve prolapse is easily evaluated by real-time scan.

<u>Radiographic findings</u>: Although not a necessary part of the usual work-up, cardiac radiographs demonstrate RV enlargement with anterior impingement of the cardiac silhouette to at least 50% of the sternum on the lateral projection. The main pulmonary artery is prominent and

interestingly, pulmonary vascular markings are usually normal if no pulmonary hypertension is present.

Cardiac cath: Classical findings demonstrate a large left to right atrial shunt with resulting high pulmonary blood flow. Pulmonary to systemic flow ratios are usually quite in excess of 2:1. Pulmonary vascular resistance is normal [in low range of 1-3 units/m^2]. Theoretically if pulmonary vascular resistance were completely normal in a patient with high pulmonary blood flow, it would be less than 1 unit/m^2. Pulmonary arteriograms on angled projections demonstrate flow of contrast material across the atrial communication.

Importantly, one must rule out associated anomalous pulmonary venous return. This is quite common in patients with sinus venosus variations of ASD. Furthermore, partial anomalous pulmonary venous return with intact atrial septum may present with identical findings of ASD, although in this group of patients the second heart sound is not as "fixed" usually.

Similar lesions physiologically: The two other most common variations of ASD are sinus venosus defects at the junction of the superior vena cava and right atrium, and ostium primum atrial septal defects [within the spectrum of endocardial cushion defects]. Sinus venosus defects differ from classical secundum ASD basically in association with a higher incidence of partial anomalous pulmonary venous return [usually on the right], and a potentially higher incidence of post operative dysrhythmia. Surgically, cannulation of the superior vena cava must be more superior, because of the defects position and care to redirect anomalous pulmonary venous return is essential.

Ostium primum ASD differs from other forms with a high association of mitral and/or tricuspid regurgitation of a variable degree. The mitral valve is cleft and the position of the ASD is quite easy to identify on echocardiography. Cath should include a left ventricular cineangiogram to evaluate the classical LV contour [goose-neck deformity] for definitive diagnosis and importantly, to evaluate mitral insufficiency. Doppler studies are very useful to non-invasively evaluate the degrees of A-V valve insufficiency.

An important physiological variation possible with ostium primum ASD is the presence of a significant left ventricular to right atrial shunt, across the cleft in the mitral valve. This form of shunt is obviously from a high to a low pressure chamber and occurs regardless of compliance or resistance differences between the right and left sides of the heart. Such shunting is commonly marked and could be associated with development of earlier pulmonary vascular disease. The presence of an associated left ventricular to right atrial shunt often requires earlier repair. The ECG in children with ostium primum ASD has a left superior QRS axis in 95% of cases and a high incidence of first degree A-V block. Findings of diastolic overload are similar to secundum ASD on precordial leads [rsR' in V1/V4R] with prominent rightward forces as well.

Other interesting causes of left to right shunts at the atrial level [increased oxygen saturation at the atrial level], include coronary arteriovenous fistula draining to right atrium, ruptured sinus of Valsalva aneurysm into right atrium, ventricular septal defect with associated tricuspid insufficiency, as well as a defect in the septum exactly between left ventricle and right atrium resulting in a direct left ventricular to right atrial shunt.

Management: Because there is little threat of pulmonary vascular disease and usually no significant compromise of growth and development, surgical closure of ASD almost becomes a social decision, relating to timing that appears good for the parent and the child. Ordinarily this means correction by 4 to 6 years of age. Although non-operative closure techniques involving catheterization placement of an umbrella have been used in selected cases, the author believes that refinement of such procedures is necessary for safety. When working without direct view of the defect, partial closure is possible and left atrial embolic phenomenon is possible as well. Certainly partial anomalous venous return would not be amenable to non-operative closure. Earlier correction would be necessary in the child with CHF that is not easily managed, as can occur in ostium primum ASD with mitral insufficiency. Postoperative long-term results are usually excellent, with only a low incidence of cardiac dysrhythmias [somewhat higher in sinus venosus group as noted above], and only a slight compromise of cardiac function if evaluated non-invasively. There is no significant decrease in functional capacity, however. All sport participation is possible if no significant dysrhythmia is present. If correction is delayed or the diagnosis missed, then the patient is at some risk of pulmonary vascular disease in which case eventual cyanosis would develop from reversal of the atrial shunt to a right to left shunt and no correction would be possible. A rare cause of cyanosis in the patient with ASD who has a normal pulmonary vascular resistance is angulation of the inferior vena cava toward an inferiorly positioned ASD with streaming of IVC return to the left atrium. Obviously, operative repair relieves cyanosis in this rare event. Prior to operative closure, the patient would require standard SBE prophylaxis. If mitral prolapse or insufficiency were present post-operatively, then SBE prophylaxis would be necessary post-operatively as well.

II. LEFT TO RIGHT SHUNTS AT THE VENTRICULAR OR GREAT VESSEL LEVEL:

Isolated Ventricular Septal Defect [VSD] and Patent Ductus Arteriosus [PDA]:

Physiology: The classical form of ventricular or pulmonary arterial left to right shunt is the uncomplicated ventricular septal defect [VSD] and patent ductus arteriosus [PDA] along with significant variations. The infant or child with uncomplicated moderate to large VSD or PDA usually manifests little in the way of physical findings until the high neonatal pulmonary vascular resistance, decreases to a lower level, between 4 to 6 weeks of age. However, in the case of small VSD or small PDA, where pressure differences can be maintained between both ventricles or both great vessels as early as the immediate newborn period, murmurs of small VSD or small PDA are present. The basic physiological consequence of VSD and of PDA is the transmission of potentially *high pressures* and *high blood flow* from the left to right ventricle [VSD] or from aorta to pulmonary artery [PDA], resulting in a very *increased pulmonary blood flow* at very *increased pressures* [see Fig. 6.4]. The magnitude of the left to right ventricular shunt or left to right pulmonary arterial shunt relates to the size of the defect, the vascular resistance ratio of the pulmonary and systemic circulations, and also in the case of VSD, the presence or absence of anatomical pulmonary stenosis.

Natural History: As with most other congenital cardiac defects, the individual patient's natural history varies according to the size of the defect. In infants and children with very large PDA or VSD, symptoms and signs of congestive cardiac failure [CHF] usually develop by 4 to 6 weeks of age, once the pulmonary vascular resistance decreases from its high newborn level to a lower level, and at a time when physiological anemias are usually responsible for relatively low oxygen carrying capacity [low hemoglobin and hematocrit levels]. The larger the defect, the worse the potential CHF, and the more maximal the anticongestive failure therapy, including digoxin,

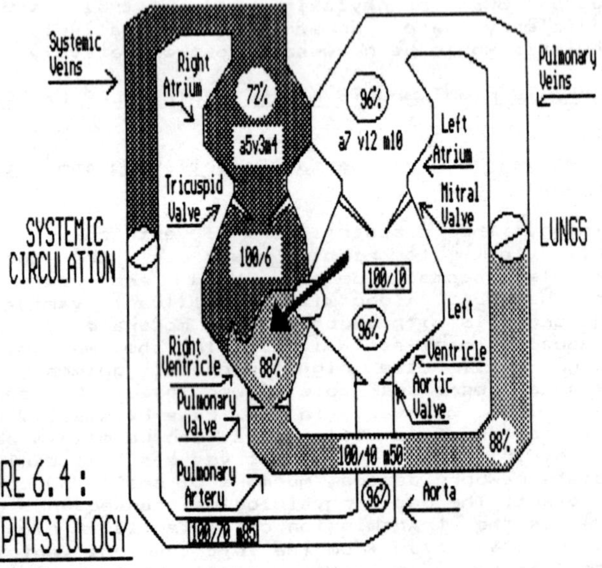

FIGURE 6.4: VSD PHYSIOLOGY

chlorothiazide or furosemide, and aldactone. Occasionally, afterload reduction with hydralazine or prazosin becomes necessary. Cardiac cachexia may result from chronic severe CHF. In moderate to small defects, natural history is ordinarily unremarkable. Mild CHF, if present at all, is usually easy to control with daily lanoxin and chlorthiazide taken every other day , or with daily lanoxin and chlorthiazide as well as aldactone. Although there is a great tendency for spontaneous closure of VSD, those defects that are large often remain open, after closing partially, and may even require surgical closure if they remain hemodynamically significant. If a small to moderate PDA has not closed by 18 months to 2 years of age, then it likely will stay open and require closure. The major threat and consequence of these high pressure, high pulmonary blood flow lesions, is the development of irreversible pulmonary vascular disease. This is a very rare event at sea level in the uncomplicated, simple VSD or PDA, before 18 months of age. However, in children with Down syndrome, even at sea level, in children with a common atrioventricular septal defect, and in children with associated complete transposition of the great vessels, development of early pulmonary vascular disease before 9 months to one year of age, is possible.

In the unusual child, the high neonatal pulmonary vascular resistance remains rather high after the neonatal period and findings of CHF or other manifestations of a large VSD or PDA are much less apparent. This group is especially important in terms of early detection and management, because these children could develop irreversible vascular disease with no previous history of significant CHF or cardiac findings.

In the moderate to small VSD, spontaneous closure often involves transient formation of a ventricular septal aneurysm. Although usually uncomplicated, rare instances of large VSD aneurysm are known. In some cases, the aneurysm may point toward the right ventricular outflow region and cause significant pulmonary stenosis. In other cases, the aneurysm may actually cross the tricuspid valve and cause a direct left ventricular right atrial pattern of left to right shunt.

A less common complication of moderate to large VSD is the evolution of associated aortic insufficiency, because of a defect's proximity with the aortic valve, with resulting weakening of the support of the aortic valve and with negative pressure developing beneath the valve from a Bernoulli phenomenon as the ventricular left to right shunt flows beneath the aortic valve in this group of patients.

In approximately 6% of children with uncomplicated VSD, significant subpulmonary [infundibular] stenosis evolves and protects the pulmonary circulation from the high pressures and high flows. If the degree of pulmonary stenosis becomes very severe, the physiology becomes similar to that of children having tetralogy of Fallot, and need for surgical intervention is more usual, even if the size of the VSD itself becomes smaller over several years.

Physical Findings: The dominant findings of VSD and PDA relate specifically to their size, hemodynamically. In the unusual circumstance of extreme VSD such as in a large common atrioventricular septal defect, common ventricle, or extremely large PDA, there may be little or no murmur at all to suggest the defect's presence. Furthermore, even with the usual large to moderate defect, murmurs may not be present until a significant left to right shunt develops across the defect upon decreasing pulmonary vascular resistance. It is quite common for a family to ask the cardiologist why the family physician failed to recognize the presence of large VSD in the neonatal nursery, and it is important to explain that significant murmurs are often not present during the immediate neonatal period.

The classical VSD murmur associated with moderate and large defects is the holosystolic, raspy murmur maximal at the lower left sternal edge with rightward radiation and slight superior radiation. If the defect is located above the crista supraventricularis, the classical murmur of VSD may be heard in a more superior location and possibly even in the left infraclavicular area. The classical PDA murmur is a continuous, raspy, "rocky," distinct murmur with maximal location at the left infraclavicular area and some radiation to the upper left sternal border as well as lateral radiation. The lateral radiation of murmurs associated with defects that augment pulmonary blood flow, such as VSD and PDA usually reflects associated physiological peripheral pulmonary stenosis secondary to the increased pulmonary blood flow.

As the VSD or PDA become smaller, the murmurs change significantly. Generally, the smaller the defect, the shorter the murmur. In the case of VSD, the murmur becomes ejection in quality and does not occupy all of systole. When very small, the murmur becomes quite short and has a definite "squirty" quality. This quality murmur is comforting in that it implies that the defect will likely close completely in the near future. The only significant serious differential to this quality murmur involves the combination of large VSD with very severe infundibular pulmonary stenosis, in which case the murmur is occasionally "squirty" as well. In this instance however, a diminished or absent pulmonary component of the second heart sound, a more forcible right ventricular impulse, possible cyanosis as well as evidence for overt RVH on the ECG would suggest the more serious combination of VSD with balanced, severe infundibular stenosis. Interestingly, when very small, a PDA may cause a short, puffy or squirty systolic ejection murmur with harsh overtones, maximal at the left infraclavicular area.

Palpation of the heart in cases of large VSD or PDA allows appreciation of mild to moderate cardiomegaly with lateral displacement of the apical impulse. The quality of the apical impulse is very hyperdynamic. When large enough to cause high right ventricular [RV] pressure, an RV lift is present at the lower left sternal border. VSD usually causes a systolic thrill at the lower left sternal border, whereas PDA is often associated with a systolic thrill in the left infraclavicular area or suprasternal notch region. The first heart sound is usually normal; however, with the holosystolic VSD murmur, it may be impossible to assess. In the case of common atrioventricular septal defect, the first heart sound is increased because of the associated mitral valve abnormalities. With PDA, the first heart sound is usually normal. The second heart sound in VSD and PDA importantly reflects the degree of pulmonary hypertension, in that significant pulmonary hypertension causes marked accentuation of the pulmonary component of the second heart sound, which also becomes more narrowly split with increased pulmonary arterial pressures and resistance. In PDA the second heart sound may rarely even become paradoxically split, whereby it becomes more wide during expiration instead of inspiration. Obviously, it is essential to carefully assess the second heart sound when there is a potential for significant pulmonary hypertension and eventual pulmonary vascular disease. Unfortunately, in the very large VSD or PDA, the length of the murmur may be such that it is not completely possible to determine the nature of the second heart sound and of its pulmonary component. A third heart sound is common in both lesions, when pulmonary blood flow is high. High pulmonary blood flow with VSD or PDA usually manifests in a mid diastolic rumble at the apex [over the mitral valve], because of increased flow across this valve, which is relatively small in relation to this increase in blood flow. Physiologically, if one hears a mid diastolic rumble, the pulmonary to systemic blood flow ratio is at least 2:1 or greater. When a VSD becomes smaller, it is common for the mid diastolic rumble to eventually disappear. One must make certain that it has not disappeared because an increased pulmonary vascular resistance has resulted in a decreased pulmonary blood flow. In this case, the intensity of the pulmonary component of the second heart sound would still be loud, reflecting the pulmonary hypertension, and the second heart sound would still be rather narrowly split.

Hepatomegaly occurs in the child with associated CHF. As previously stated, one must carefully assess the quality of the liver edge, because low grade chronic CHF may manifest in a dull liver edge with no overt clinical enlargement of the liver.

Pulses in patients with VSD are usually prominent because of an associated rapid upstroke of the pulse. In cases of PDA, pulses are very full volume, resulting in a description of "bounding." It is often possible to palpate the dorsalis pedis and posterior tibial pulses even through thin socks in such infants and children, not that this should be evaluated in such a manner.

Differential Diagnosis: The major differential diagnosis of the VSD murmur at the lower left sternal border would be tricuspid insufficiency, which may occur transiently in the newborn. This murmur however, is usually described as more blowing and superficial in quality. A traumatic delivery or one associated with transient hypoxemia in the newborn, should alert the examining physician to the possibility of tricuspid insufficiency associated with a persistent high pulmonary vascular resistance. The major differential of the continuous PDA murmur would be a similar murmur associated with aortico-pulmonary window. Other continuous murmurs include those associated with coronary arterio-venous malformations and aberrant left coronary artery, but in these instances, the more distinct component of the continuous murmur would be diastolic and not systolic, because coronary flow is a diastolic event, essentially. Older literature states that the combination of VSD murmur with that of aortic insufficiency might appear continuous. However, the author usually finds this combination of murmurs quite distinct and not continuous in quality.

ECG Findings: Once out of the immediate newborn period, when RVH is possible, large VSD and PDA usually causes biventricular hypertrophy or at least left ventricular hypertrophy. Left atrial abnormality is common, and the frontal axis is normal or somewhat leftward. As with other forms of endocardial cushion defect, common atrioventricular septal defect generally manifests a left [or occasionally a right] superior QRS axis. Double outlet right ventricle also manifests such a superior QRS axis, but with less frequency. Interestingly, children with large VSD associated with complete transposition of the great vessels also often display a left superior QS axis on ECG. As the VSD becomes smaller, spontaneously, evidence for ventricular hypertrophy and left atrial abnormality becomes less. If pulmonary vascular disease or significant pulmonary stenosis develops, RVH becomes apparent.

ECHO Findings: In the majority of patients with significant VSD, the ECHO is able to document the position and extent of the defect. The one exception involves the inferior muscular septal regions where multiple VSDs are possible and may not be visualized. Newer technology using color mapped Doppler techniques may prove useful in this group of patients.

In children with large to moderate PDA, the vessel is usually directly visualized on several cross-sectional ECHO projections. Doppler evaluation is also useful. Findings of left ventricular and left atrial enlargement would be expected in both VSD and PDA, if moderate or large.

Radiographic Findings: Radiographic findings are not specific for VSD or PDA but rather reflect an increased pulmonary blood flow. In the case of large defects, evidence for CHF is possible, including cardiomegaly. Main pulmonary arterial prominence is possible when pulmonary hypertension is present with increased pulmonary blood flow. Left ventricular and left atrial prominence are common.

Cardiac Cath: Definitive diagnosis by cardiac cath is still suggested in order to assess the status of pulmonary vascular resistance and the exact anatomical location of VSD. Administration of oxygen and tolazoline might be necessary in the child with long standing VSD or PDA when a question of operability arises because of possible irreversible pulmonary vascular disease. Cath is ordinarily suggested in the older child with PDA, although in the instance of moderate to small PDA in the older child with no evidence for significant pulmonary hypertension and with ECHO demonstration of the usual position for PDA, it is likely that surgical ligation without cath will become more popular. Detection of associated aortic insufficiency or pulmonary stenosis, in the case of VSD, is important.

Similar Lesions Physiologically: The most similar lesion to uncomplicated VSD is double outlet right ventricle [DORV] with subpulmonary VSD, in which case, apart from slight systemic desaturation, physical and physiological findings are similar. A left superior QRS axis on the ECG and the ECHO ordinarily allow this diagnosis prior to cardiac cath. Surgically, it is essential that the surgeon is aware of this variation so as not to patch the VSD as usual, but to direct left ventricular ejection to the aorta via a tunnel like patch, making certain that the VSD itself is large enough. Restriction at the ventricular septal defect level, would behave physiologically as aortic stenosis in these patients.

Another important physiological variant of VSD is common atrioventricular septal defect [common A-V Canal], with associated varying degrees of atrio-ventricular valve insufficiency. ECHO and Doppler are excellent non-invasive methods to determine the exact configuration of the atrio-ventricular valves, including any problems with override, straddling, or insufficiency. An interesting variant physiologically is direct left ventricular - right atrial shunting which occurs regardless of the ratio of pulmonary to systemic vascular resistances. Marked degrees of straddling of the A-V valves in these patients occasionally results in underdevelopment of one ventricle, rendering early correction impossible, surgically.

The major physiological variant of PDA is the aortico-pulmonary window, located between the ascending aorta and pulmonary artery, not the descending aorta. Newer ECHO imaging techniques should differentiate aortico-pulmonary window from uncomplicated PDA. However, definitive cath diagnosis is still likely to be safer in cases of suspected aortico-pulmonary window, because the surgical approach is so different [mid sternotomy compared with left thoracotomy]. Importantly, these cases involve very large defects, and the necessity to differentiate small PDA from aortico-pulmonary window is slight.

Management: There are two basic issues relating to sensible management of high pressure, high flow lesions such as VSD and PDA. The most important issue in VSD management is timing of surgical closure relative to development of irreversible pulmonary vascular disease. A limited number of surgical centers have eradicated age related mortality and morbidity, so that surgical closure is possible at very early ages. Ordinarily, if one does not encounter significant CHF, closure of a significant defect between 6 to 9 months of age is reasonable. Potential threat of irreversible vascular disease in uncomplicated VSD at sea level is rare before 18 months of age. However if the patient has a more complex form, such as A-V canal or the infant has Down Syndrome, pulmonary vascular disease can occur between 6 to 9 months, and persistence of high pressure and high flow into the pulmonary circulation should not be allowed beyond that time in such patients. If anatomy is extremely complex and anticipated mortality and morbidity is therefore much higher than usual, some medical centers would still prefer to perform palliative surgery involving placement of a pulmonary arterial band to decrease flow and pressure seen by the pulmonary circulation. This procedure does not ensure against development of irreversible pulmonary vascular disease if the band is too loose and might not be tolerated if the band is too tight. Furthermore, this procedure should not be attempted in children with left ventricular to right atrial shunts. This high to low pressure shunt would persist even after banding which would not be tolerated.

Similar guidelines apply in large PDA. In smaller PDA, one can safely wait for possible spontaneous closure until 1 year to 18 months of age.

The second most important management decision in patients with VSD is safe postponement of any surgical intervention to allow spontaneous closure. Generally if pulmonary arterial pressures are less than 1/2 systemic levels, the threat of irreversible pulmonary vascular disease is small. In such patients, it is usually safe to wait beyond 18 months if cath indicates no significant increase in pulmonary vascular resistance. The majority of small VSDs will close spontaneously by 1 year of age or soon thereafter. In patients followed for the moderate defects as above, repeat cardiac cath unfortunately becomes necessary to make certain that no pulmonary vascular disease is present. After adequate follow up, if pulmonary arterial pressures are normal and pulmonary to systemic blood flow ratios are less than 1.2-1.4:1.0, one is usually able to safely make a decision to follow the patient indefinitely without plans for surgery. Should significant aortic insufficiency or subpulmonary stenosis develop, surgical intervention is almost always necessary.

Many patients with small membranous VSD have spontaneous closure of the defect by formation of a transient ventricular septal aneurysm. Such aneurysms still require SBE prophylaxis and are suspected clinically by appreciation of a systolic click at the mid sternal border. SBE prophylaxis would not be necessary in patients undergoing spontaneous VSD closure without VSD aneurysm formation. Similarly such prophylaxis is not necessary longer than 6 months after spontaneous or surgical closure of PDA.

III. LARGE VSD WITH SIGNIFICANT PULMONARY STENOSIS:

Physiology: The classical form of this physiological group of lesions is tetralogy of Fallot, which by definition includes the VSD, severe pulmonary stenosis, in addition to right ventricular hypertrophy and aortic override of the ventricular septum. The determinant of physiological severity of the combination of pulmonary stenosis and large VSD relates to a constant balance between the right ventricular ejection pathway impedance and the impedance and vascular resistance faced by the left ventricular ejection pathway. The higher the impedance in the right ventricular ejection pathway relative to the impedance and afterload of the left ventricular ejection pathway, the more desirable it is for the right ventricle to eject more volume [at systemic mixed venous saturation] toward the left ventricular ejection path and subsequently into the aorta [see Fig. 6.5]. The RV obstruction [impedance] may be very dynamic in the form of infundibular muscular narrowing and distortion, or relatively fixed in the form of severe pulmonary valvar or supravalvar stenosis. The extreme variation of this physiology involves pulmonary valve atresia, in which case physiology then becomes common mixing physiology and patent ductus arteriosus dependent. Should the PDA close in such an instance there would be no path for flow to reach the pulmonary circulation and the infant could not survive. Prostaglandin therapy would be necessary in the immediate newborn period should this occur.

The other end of the interesting spectrum of this physiological group is the acyanotic child with a perfect balance between RV ejection path impedance and LV ejection path impedance and afterload, resulting in a minimal or no shunt from RV to the aorta, across the VSD.

Natural History: Clinical course relates to the severity of the pulmonary stenosis, basically. As noted in the physiology discussion, a small group of infants suffer from the extreme variation involving pulmonary atresia and require stabilization with prostaglandin therapy and neonatal palliative procedures such as aortico-pulmonary arterial anastomosis. With lesser degrees of pulmonary stenosis the infant could remain completely asymptomatic until several years of age. Risk of hypercyanotic spells occurs in the moderate to severe pulmonary stenosis group [see discussion of hypercyanotic spell physiology and therapy in Cardiac Emergency chapter].

It is important to emphasize that this group of lesions is not associated with congestive cardiac failure, and if one makes such a diagnosis in a patient said to have large VSD

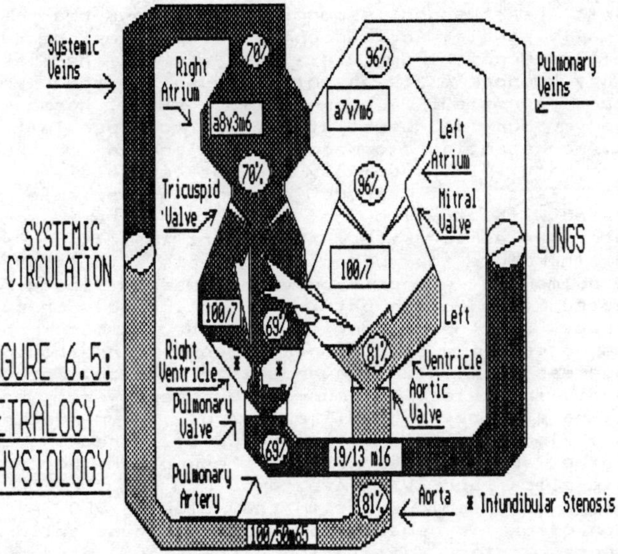

FIGURE 6.5: TETRALOGY PHYSIOLOGY

and severe pulmonary stenosis, then one has to question the anatomical diagnosis. This group of lesions represents a spectrum of cyanotic congenital heart disease from the severely cyanotic infant to the nearly acyanotic, relative to the degree of pulmonary stenosis. Increasing degrees of pulmonary stenosis causes increasing degrees of cyanosis. In general, the "wellness" of the child depends almost directly on the total pulmonary blood flow. The more the pulmonary blood flow, the more oxygenated blood that is available to enter the aorta. It is logical that palliative approaches attempt to augment the total pulmonary blood flow.

Physical Findings: The easiest way to elaborate the usual physical findings in the entire spectrum of these lesions is first to describe findings of classical tetralogy of Fallot. The infant on general exam is usually adequately developed and nourished, and in no distress. The apical impulse is not displaced and is not hyperdynamic. There is a significant RV heave at the lower left sternal border. The first heart sound is normal. The second heart sound is classically single, not accentuated and best heard at the mid left sternal border in lieu of at the base [the pulmonary component is absent because of the severity of pulmonary stenosis]. A non-specific, short, harsh systolic ejection murmur is present at the mid to upper left sternal border, representing forward flow along an obstructed RV ejection path. Interestingly and not completely understood is the fact that there are no appreciable murmurs associated with the flow of blood from the RV across the VSD into the aorta [i.e., the right to left intracardiac shunt]. Therefore the murmur in patients with large VSD and severe pulmonary stenosis only represents flow across the obstructed RV ejection path. When following such patients, a decrease in the intensity of the murmur represents increasing severity of pulmonary stenosis and should prompt more aggressive evaluation and intervention. Occasionally the systolic ejection murmur becomes very "squirty," suggesting a closing VSD, but truly representing flow across a long segment of infundibular narrowing. In such cases, the abnormal second heart sound, the presence of a systolic click and RV heave, and RVH on the ECG should point to a more serious lesion than closing VSD. A systolic ejection click is usually present in these children and represents aortic dilatation from the increased flow contributed by the RV. The severity of pulmonary stenosis is so great that a click from the pulmonary valve is unlikely.

On the other end of the spectrum is the child with excellent balance of pulmonary stenosis and large VSD. In such cases one may appreciate prominent splitting of the second heart sound with a decreased but nevertheless audible pulmonary component. Loss of the pulmonary component in this group indicates increasing severity of pulmonary stenosis. In this group also, one might appreciate a VSD quality murmur if any flow occurs from left to right ventricle across the VSD.

In the extremely cyanotic infant with this group of lesions, it is common for no murmur to be present. All one then appreciates is the singular nature of the second heart sound, the systolic click, and the RV heave.

Differential Diagnosis: Another form of cyanotic congenital heart disease that could be confused with these lesions is tricuspid atresia complex with associated severe pulmonary stenosis; however, echocardiography easily differentiates these patients.

A very interesting variant in anatomy involves fibrous stenosis of the ostium infundibulum or the inlet of the infundibular chamber. This defect is occasionally listed under double chamber right ventricle. Anomalous right ventricular muscle bundles may also cause rather proximal stenosis within the RV, but are usually not associated with VSD. If a large VSD is present with stenosis of the ostium infundibulum, then physiology becomes that of tetralogy of Fallot. Cardiac catheterization ordinarily separates these variations.

ECG Findings: RVH is the rule with pure R waves in leads V1/ V4R and/or upright T waves in these leads. One other observation is that inferior forces [R waves in leads II/III/AVF] are often prominent. If the child has a variant involving endocardial cushion defect or double outlet RV, there would most often be a left superior frontal QRS axis [> -30 to -45 degrees].

ECHO Findings: Exact diagnosis by echocardiography is possible in this group of lesions with excellent definition of the VSD and malalignment of a dilated aortic root. The level of pulmonary stenosis is usually possible to assess as is the size of the proximal pulmonary arteries. One thing that remains difficult is the determination of multiple levels of pulmonary arterial stenoses, peripherally. If open, a PDA is usually easy to identify as well.

Radiographic Findings: Classically one observes a normal cardiothoracic ratio, upturning of the apex, consistent with RV enlargement, a decreased pulmonary artery segment, and decreased pulmonary vascular markings. The overall impression is that the cardiac silhouette resembles a "boot." The more diminished the pulmonary blood flow the more oligemic the lung fields become. In 25% of patients, one identifies a right aortic arch.

Cardiac Cath: Important reasons for continuing to perform cardiac cath in these patients are to definitively outline the level and severity of pulmonary stenosis, to demonstrate pulmonary arterial configuration and size, to consider additional VSDs, and to assess coronary arterial configuration [it is not uncommon to find a conal branch of the coronary arteries coursing horizontally along the infundibular region, making incisions in this region impossible]. Newer techniques involving resection of the infundibular narrowing by establishing exposure from across the tricuspid valve, avoids the RV incision, often.

Similar Lesions Physiologically: Important anatomical variations that behave almost identically, physiologically, include complete atrioventricular septal defect with severe pulmonary stenosis. In such cases variable degrees of A-V valve insufficiency complicate the physiology and closure of the VSD becomes more difficult, technically. As noted above, a left superior axis on the ECG suggests this variant or double outlet RV. In the instance of double outlet RV with severe pulmonary stenosis, echocardiography and angiography enable accurate diagnosis. One is able to appreciate distribution of conal tissue beneath both semilunar valves in that each is at the same horizontal level. It is critical for the surgeon to appreciate this variation of anatomy so that the left ventricular ejection pathway remains widely open as the VSD is patched to the aorta in such a way to preserve unobstructed LV ejection. Simple closure of the VSD in these patients would obliterate any LV ejection path and result in demise of the patient.

Common ventricle [no ventricular septum at all] or univentricular configurations with associated severe pulmonary stenosis also require careful surgical consideration. Total correction in this group could involve variations of tricuspid atresia surgery, or the Fontan operation.

Stenosis of the ostium infundibulum with large VSD is another interesting variant [see differential diagnosis above].

Management: Timing for total surgical correction relates to the severity of pulmonary stenosis forcing early intervention and the presence of any more serious defects such as complete atrioventricular septal defect or double outlet RV. Timing also relates to the experience in a given medical center. Certain outstanding centers and their surgeons have eradicated an age related mortality and morbidity for these patients, who may undergo total correction in infancy if necessary. More often, if an anatomically complicated form of these lesions exists and the infant requires early intervention when less than 6 months to 1 year of age, then a surgeon would perform a palliative procedure involving an aortico-pulmonary anastomosis. The classic form of such a procedure if the Blalock-Taussig anastomosis or shunt whereby the subclavian artery is connected to the ipsilateral pulmonary artery. Blood flow to the upper extremity is preserved by collateral circulation although pulses are usually absent after the procedure. One usually first chooses the subclavian artery associated with the innominate or brachiocephalic artery which is the first aortic arch vessel. In the usual left aortic arch, this would be the right subclavian artery. In the case of right aortic arch, this would be the left subclavian artery. Pre-operative cath assessment of possible anomalous subclavian is obviously critical for such surgery.

A newer option to the Blalock-Taussig shunt is interposition of at least a 4-5 mm Goretex tubular graft between the ipsilateral subclavian and pulmonary artery. One must make certain that these shunts are restrictive to pressure and yet allow adequate augmentation of pulmonary blood flow. It was fortuitous that the original choice of subclavian vessels was so perfect in this regard. Larger vessels or shunts could allow increases in pulmonary arterial pressure and enough increase in pulmonary blood flow to cause CHF.

Total repair of these defects often results in pulmonary insufficiency and complete right bundle branch block, which are usually well tolerated, indefinitely.

It is important to realize that continued presence of very small pulmonary arteries after many years may make any total correction impossible.

IV. COMPLETE TRANSPOSITION OF THE GREAT VESSELS [D-LOOP/D-TGV]:

Physiology: The basic physiological problem with complete transposition of the great vessels [D-Loop,D-Transposition] is the presence of two independent parallel circulations in lieu of series circulations as is normal. Because the aorta arises from the right ventricle which receives systemic venous return from the right atrium, systemic venous return recirculates into the systemic circulation. Because the pulmonary artery arises directly from the left ventricle which receives pulmonary venous return from the left atrium, pulmonary venous return recirculates into the pulmonary circulation. It should be apparent that survival is not possible unless a communication exists between these two parallel circulations, allowing a flow of saturated pulmonary venous return into the systemic circulation and allowing a flow of desaturated systemic venous return into the pulmonary circulation. Furthermore, net flow from one parallel side must equal net flow to the other parallel side, otherwise one side would empty its volume into the other [see Fig. 6.6]. The physiological flow crossing between both parallel circulations is the effective pulmonary blood flow, which is essentially the most important flow to calculate in these children. It reflects how well mixing is occurring between both circulations. The definition of right to left shunt remains the same and is the net flow of blood with mixed systemic venous saturation that enters the systemic circulation. Hence, with transposition, it is the amount of blood flow that recirculates in the systemic part of the two parallel circulations. Similarly, the left to right shunt is the amount of blood flow that recirculates in the pulmonary part of the two parallel circulations.

Sites of usual admixture of pulmonary and systemic venous returns usually involve an atrial septal defect. If one is not present at birth then a balloon atrial septostomy must be performed as soon as possible. Other sites of admixture include ventricular septal defects and patent ductus arteriosus. In the latter regard, administration of prostaglandin E_1 could be very helpful in the initial management of the markedly hypoxic neonate with inadequate effective pulmonary blood flow. It would promote temporary PDA patency to allow another site of mixing, until performance of a balloon atrial septostomy.

Natural History: The usual course of infants with complete transposition varies according to the associated defects. In the infant with a successful balloon atrial septostomy and no other lesions such as VSD or pulmonary stenosis, a period of marked stability occurs after the immediate newborn period and usually until the time of corrective surgery which should be performed no later than 6 to 9 months of age, because of the great risk of early development of pulmonary vascular disease, after 6 months of age, even without associated VSD or other high pressure lesions. Newer surgical techniques allow "arterial swith" in the immediate newborn period with no balloon atrial septostomy, depending upon exact anatomy.

In the infant with large VSD, although mixing is usually adequate, the further presence of high pressure in an extremely high pulmonary blood flow lesion results in early congestive cardiac failure. If this is not easily

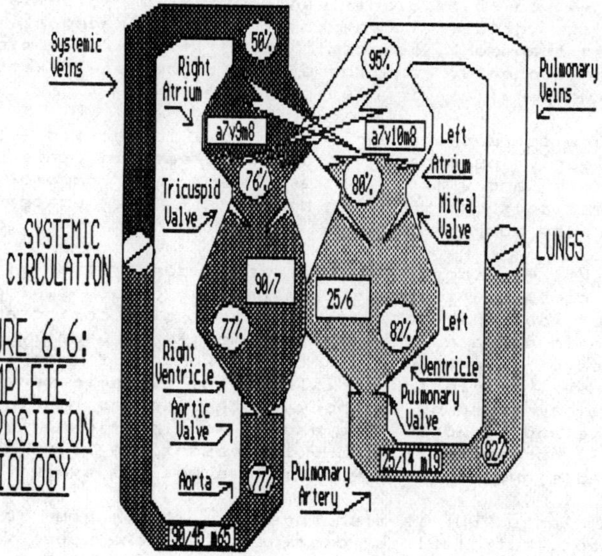

FIGURE 6.6: COMPLETE TRANSPOSITION PHYSIOLOGY

manageable, total surgical correction may be the only option. If this is not possible because of other unusual problems such as underdevelopment of a ventricle associated with a common atrioventricular septal defect, then pulmonary arterial banding may be the only form of palliation available in early infancy.

A small subgroup of infants will display inadequate mixing even after adequate balloon atrial septostomy. Depending upon a particular center's experience either total surgical correction or surgical creation of an atrial septal defect would help such infants.

Generally, one follows these infants carefully for signs of significant hypoxia such as tachypnea, dyspnea or hyperpnea. Although arterial oxygen tensions may be as low as 35-40 Torr, adequacy of oxygenation is noted by normal acid base balance [i.e., normal range base excess, no less than -4 to -5]. Significant metabolic acidemia with base deficits greater than -5 indicate inadequate systemic oxygen transport [systemic blood flow x systemic arterial oxygen content], and therefore inadequate mixing between the two parallel circulations.

Failure to perform early surgical correction could allow very early pulmonary vascular disease in this group of patients and many centers are now promoting total correction shortly after birth, if the anatomy is not otherwise complicated.

Physical Findings: The classical description of an infant with complete transposition and no other lesions such as VSD or pulmonary stenosis, is that of a comfortable deeply cyanotic neonate. The apical impulse is usually normal. An RV heave is present at the lower left sternal border because the right ventricle is the systemic ventricle. The first heart sound is normal; the second heart sound is single and loud at the base. No significant murmurs are usually present. If no CHF is present the liver is normally palpable and pulses are normal as well as symmetrical.

If a large VSD is also present, the murmur of VSD is present, but is less distinct than the usual VSD murmur. The second heart sound may appear split. Because the pulmonary valve is so far posterior, the pulmonary component would not be accentuated to reflect the significant pulmonary hypertension.

With both VSD and significant pulmonary stenosis, findings begin to mimic those of tetralogy of Fallot, although systolic clicks are not common in patients with transposition.

Differential Diagnosis: The most significant differential diagnosis involves tetralogy of Fallot and common mixing lesions such as truncus arteriosus. In the case of tetralogy, a systolic click is usually present and the second heart sound is not accentuated, although it is single. Radiographs of the chest display oligemic lung fields with tetralogy and increased pulmonary blood flow with transposition. With truncus, a systolic click and loud single second heart sound are present. The precordium is usually much more hyperdynamic with truncus compared with uncomplicated complete transposition, and the patient is ordinarily less cyanotic with truncus.

ECG Findings: RVH is usually present. With associated VSD the frontal QRS axis is usually in the left superior range, similar to patients with endocardial cushion defects.

ECHO Findings: Cross-sectional imaging adequately demonstrates the pulmonary artery arising from the left ventricle and the aorta arising from the right ventricle. Additional lesions such as large VSD, PDA, ASD, pulmonary or subpulmonary stenosis are easily elaborated as well. Some centers with good experience are now performing balloon atrial septostomies in the newborn nursery under cross-sectional guidance. The exact form of subpulmonary stenosis often present in these patients is also well displayed by ECHO.

Radiographic Findings: Classically there is an apparent absence of thymic shadow in the newborn, likely from stress. The pulmonary vascular markings are usually increased unless significant pulmonary stenosis is present. There is a round appearance to the cardiac silhouette which is often not too enlarged. The usual pulmonary arterial arc segment is not present, resulting in a narrow "waist."

Cardiac Cath: Diagnostic cath is often not necessary because ECHO and Doppler studies are adequate to outline anatomy. However, in complex forms of complete transposition including subpulmonary stenosis, VSD, common atrioventricular septal defect, cineangiographic delineation is important. Definition of the coronary arteries is necessary when the arterial switch operation is contemplated [Jatene procedure].

Balloon atrial septostomy is critical in the newborn. If creation of an atrial communication is necessary after 1 to 2 months of age, the atrial septum is ordinarily too fibrous at that time and balloon septostomy is not possible. In these few cases, blade atrial septostomy is possible in centers with such experience. Often total surgical correction is possible, alternatively.

Similar Lesions Physiologically: Complete transposition physiology is quite unique and rarely do other anatomical defects result in such physiology. The one exception is double outlet right ventricle [DORV] with subpulmonary VSD, in which case LV ejection is directed primarily to the pulmonary circulation resulting in transposition physiology. ECHO may outline this complex lesion, but cineangiograms are essential to its complete elaboration.

Management: As noted above, many centers are now capable of performing total operative correction in patients with complete transposition in the first several weeks or months of age. In simple transposition, basically three approaches to correction are possible, depending upon the individual surgeons experience:

[1] Mustard procedure with redirection of the systemic and pulmonary venous returns at the atrial level by placement of an interatrial baffle [tunnel shaped usually from woven dacron].

[2] Senning procedure with redirection of the pulmonary and systemic venous returns using complex incisions into the native atria. Subsequent suture placement results in redirection of blood flows using the patient's own atrial tissue and no artificial material.

[3] Jatene procedure with switch of the aortic and pulmonary roots allowing for coronary arterial origin from the new aortic root and allowing for great vessel size discrepancies by special geometrical incisions of the respective vessel roots.

If any delay beyond 6 to 9 months of age is necessary because of other associated lesions, then one must be certain that the pulmonary circulation is protected with either innate pulmonary stenosis or a pulmonary arterial band.

Infants with associated large VSD and severe pulmonary stenosis often require palliative shunts as in tetralogy of Fallot [see discussion under tetralogy of Fallot].

It also important to point out that some centers are willing to perform total correction of this lesion or of tetralogy of Fallot without using any blood products. Although performed this way originally to satisfy some parents' religious convictions, at least one of these centers reports equal or slightly improved results of these operations if compared with the same group of operations when using blood products.

V. COMMON MIXING LESIONS WITH AND WITHOUT SIGNIFICANT PULMONARY STENOSIS:

Physiology: Classical examples of common mixing lesions include tricuspid atresia, total anomalous pulmonary venous return, and truncus arteriosus. In each case, there is total admixture of the pulmonary and the systemic venous returns at some point in the circulation. In the case of tricuspid atresia, all of the systemic and pulmonary venous returns must mix at the atrial level, because there is no

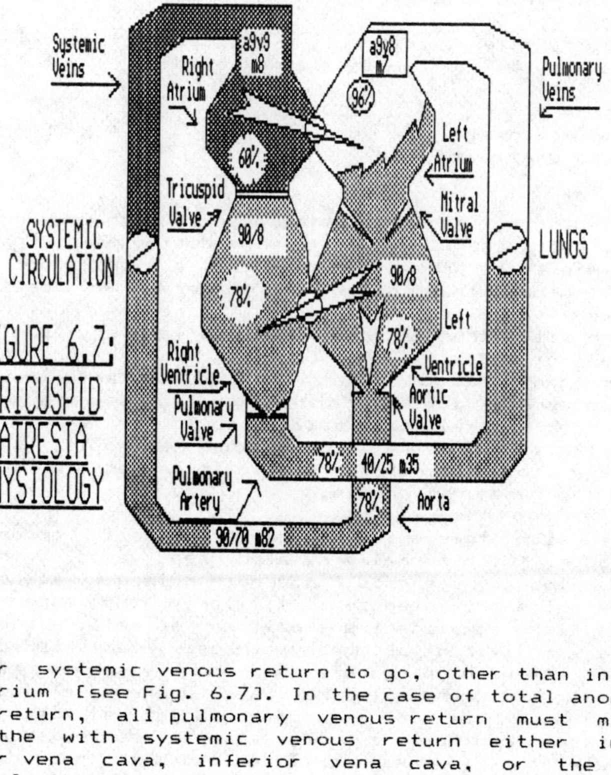

FIGURE 6.7: TRICUSPID ATRESIA PHYSIOLOGY

path for systemic venous return to go, other than into the left atrium [see Fig. 6.7]. In the case of total anomalous venous return, all pulmonary venous return must mix in common the with systemic venous return either in the superior vena cava, inferior vena cava, or the right atrium. In the case of truncus arteriosus, all systemic and pulmonary venous returns mix in the single vessel arising from the ventricles which must be joined by a large VSD. Certainly there could be some preferential streaming across the VSD into the pulmonary artery if it arises close to the truncal root [Type I truncus], but basic common mixing physiology still applies.

Interestingly, although the lesions described above are quite complex, cyanosis need not be marked if the pulmonary to systemic blood flow ratio is high. Table 6.1 demonstrates the potentially high oxygen saturation in patients with this physiology, provided the Qp/Qs is very increased. Results assume a pulmonary venous saturation of 95% and a mixed systemic venous saturation of 65%.

Table 6.1: Systemic arterial oxygen saturation versus Qp/Qs in common mixing lesions

Qp/Qs	0.5	1.0	1.5	2.0	2.5	3.0
Systemic Arterial Oxygen saturation	75	80	83	85	86.4	87.5

Natural History: Course varies according to the individual lesion, but generally, in the immediate newborn period, little might be present to suggest a significant cardiac defect, other than slight to moderate cyanosis. When pulmonary vascular resistance decreases postnatally, children with truncus arteriosus suffer very serious and often uncontrollable CHF. CHF in fact may even occur earlier than usual in infants with truncus arteriosus. With innate stenosis at the origin of the pulmonary artery from the truncal vessel, the patient could be stable almost indefinitely, unless increasing stenosis decreased pulmonary blood enough to result in marked hypoxemia with marked increase in cyanosis.

Children with tricuspid atresia are usually grouped into six groups. With normally related great vessels, there may be no pulmonary stenosis, moderate pulmonary stenosis, or extreme pulmonary stenosis; similarly the same may be present with complete transposition as well. In children with no significant pulmonary stenosis, early CHF develops as soon as the high neonatal pulmonary vascular resistance decreases. Children with moderate degrees of pulmonary stenosis may have such a good physiological balance that they appear minimally cyanotic and manifest no significant CHF. Detection in these children is often delayed beyond the neonatal period. Children with associated extreme pulmonary stenosis are usually so cyanotic that early detection is usual and a pulmonary to arterial shunt becomes necessary very early.

Infants with total anomalous pulmonary venous return [TAPVR] are often stable for several days or weeks after birth but eventually manifest symptoms of CHF with dyspnea, hyperpnea, diaphoresis, etc. Those with return below the diaphragm are at high risk of pulmonary venous obstruction, causing extreme hypoxia from decreased pulmonary blood flow and an emergent situation in regard to diagnosis and surgery.

Common to all of these lesions is the fact that the less cyanotic the patient, the higher the pulmonary to systemic blood flow ratio and the greater chance of associated CHF. With a decreased pulmonary to systemic blood flow ratio, marked cyanosis is present and intervention essential.

Physical Findings: No very specific findings are present in children with tricuspid atresia and the findings are generally those of associated degrees of pulmonary stenosis in which case the second heart sound would be prominently split with a decreased pulmonary component or single and decreased. Precordial palpation is also non-specific. If no pulmonary stenosis is present and the pulmonary blood flow is high, then the precordium would be very hyperdynamic.

Children with truncus arteriosus usually have a very hyperdynamic precordium with accentuation of both LV and RV impulses. The first heart sound is normal. The second heart sound is single and loud. Some literature describes the possible appreciation of multiple second heart sounds because of the presence of more than four cusps of the semilunar truncal valve in some patients. Typically a prominent systolic ejection click is present along the sternal border or base, reflecting dilatation of the truncus and/or the abnormal truncal valve itself. Third heart sounds and mid diastolic rumbles at the apex are common when pulmonary blood flow is increased. Although a murmur of VSD is present, it is less distinct than usual. Pulses are very full volume and often suggest PDA. Hepatomegaly depends upon the degree of CHF.

A hyperdynamic RV and widely split second heart sound may be the only findings of total anomalous venous return, in addition to a mid-diastolic rumble and third heart sound at the lower left sternal border. Marked degrees of cyanosis indicate probable obstruction to pulmonary venous return in this group of patients.

Differential Diagnosis: Depending upon associated lesions, tricuspid atresia could mimic large VSD or tetralogy of Fallot, or complete transposition. Truncus arteriosus could mimic large VSD or tetralogy of Fallot depending upon the presence of associated stenosis of the pulmonary arterial origins. Total anomalous pulmonary venous return could be mistaken for almost any other cyanotic lesion, if one fails to recognize the wide splitting of the second heart sound.

ECG Findings: Biventricular hypertrophy as well as possible biatrial abnormalities are common in truncus arteriosus.

Right axis deviation and RVH is usual for total anomalous pulmonary venous return.

Left axis deviation and LVH are typical for tricuspid atresia with associated normally related great vessels. A more normal frontal axis is present when complete transposition is also present. It is usually stated that left superior frontal QRS axis with LVH in a cyanotic newborn indicates tricuspid atresia. Right atrial abnormality is present, most often.

ECHO Findings: Delineation of truncus arteriosus and of tricuspid atresia is most often possible by cross sectional ECHO. In the case of TAPVR, it is occasionally very difficult to be certain of the diagnosis. In centers with large experience and particularly talented echocardiographers, definition of the exact form of total anomalous pulmonary venous return is often possible. Small left atrial size and absent typical drainage of pulmonary veins to the left atrium suggest this anomaly, even if the common pulmonary venous trunk is not imaged.

Radiographic Findings: Cardiomegaly, right aortic arch [in 25% of patients], left atrial enlargement, and increased pulmonary vascular markings are typical of truncus arteriosus.

Patterns of pulmonary edema are present in the neonate with obstructed pulmonary venous return. In older children the detection of a typical "snow man" appearance of the superior mediastinum from anomalous drainage of pulmonary veins to the SVC is typical. Importantly, TAPVR is a lesion where florid CHF may be present and there might not be evidence cf overt cardiomegaly on radiograph of the chest because of obstructed pulmonary venous return and resulting underloading of the central cardiac circulation.

The cardiac silhouette in the typical form of tricuspid atresia has been likened to an "apple on a stick". Right atrial enlargement and increased pulmonary vascular marking are typical if pulmonary stenosis is not severe. With increasing degrees of pulmonary stenosis, pulmonary vascular markings become decrease.

Cardiac Cath: Diagnostic cath is usually essential for TAPVR in order to completely outline the course of anomalous return. Pulmonary arteriograms allow this definition. With obstruction to pulmonary venous return, the added burden of hyperosmolar contrast material may promote worsening pulmonary edema and one should consider the newer anionic contrast materials as an alternative for these studies. Balloon atrial septostomy would be performed if the atrial septum is restrictive and total repair might be delayed. However, atrial communications in these patients are usually very large and there is some added risk to the performance of balloon atrial septostomy in this group because of the small left atrium.

Diagnostic cath is also essential in truncus arteriosus to specifically outline the pulmonary arterial origins, determine pulmonary arterial pressures, define coronary arterial anatomy, and assess the degree of truncal insufficiency, which is often present in these children. Although important it is not essential to exquisitely define the VSD which is easy to assess by ECHO. Multiple VSDs are possible but would be found at the time of surgery if missed at cath. Most surgeons would nevertheless prefer pre-operative definition of multiple VSD's. There is a significant risk of complete heart block with demise at the time of cath, and one should avoid sensitive regions of the ventricular septum during cath.

Diagnosis of tricuspid atresia is completely possible by ECHO; however, cardiac cath should be performed prior to surgical correction to make certain that pulmonary arterial pressures are low and total correction is therefore possible. If palliative shunts are necessary because of severe associated pulmonary stenosis, definition of the brachiocephalic vessels is important. Assessment of the adequacy of pulmonary arterial bands in the group with no pulmonary stenosis at birth is also important by cardiac cath.

Similar Lesions Physiologically: Hypoplastic left heart syndrome is a common mixing lesion but here inadequate systemic perfusion with poor pulses usually allows one to suspect this group of defects. For further discussion of these lesions refer to the chapter on cardiac emergencies relating to PDA dependent lesions. Pulmonary atresia with large VSD is also a common mixing lesion but is the extreme end of the spectrum of tetralogy physiology and usually considered in that group. Isolated mitral atresia with large ASD and VSD is also a common mixing lesion but so rare as not to warrant long discussion. It would be detected by ECHO, easily.

Management: Early total surgical correction is the usual rule for TAPVR. Surgical risk is greatest in the group with drainage below the diaphragm associated with obstruction. Management of CHF before surgery is obviously necessary if surgery is delayed.

Early total correction of truncus arteriosus is also necessary because of the predictable failure to thrive. When each pulmonary artery arises separately from the ascending truncus [Types II/III], total repair is more complicated but nevertheless possible. Because surgical skills are available for performing early total correction of this group of lesions, there is little place for pulmonary arterial banding unless uncontrollable CHF does not permit transfer to a center where total correction may be done with acceptable mortality and morbidity.

With tricuspid atresia and normally related great vessels, total physiological repair is possible with connection of the right atrial appendage to the pulmonary arteries, closure of the atrial septal defect and isolation of the main pulmonary artery [Fontan procedure]. Pulmonary vascular resistance must be low for safe and successful total correction. Therefore, neonatal correction is not possible using this technique. Often repair is postponed if the child is stable to between 1 and 4 years of age. Long term results appear excellent and it is fascinating that the right atrium can provide enough impulse to perfuse the pulmonary circulation. The post operative period is often complicated by significant post-pericardiotomy syndrome and physiological readjustment involving decreased systemic venous return, but eventual complete recovery is the general result. The complicated addition of complete transposition of the great vessels requires individual approaches to total physiological correction, but remains potentially correctable as well.

VI. OBSTRUCTIVE LESIONS AT THE LEVEL OF THE SEMILUNAR VALVES AND RELATED LEVELS OF OBSTRUCTION:

Physiology: The major consequence of valvar aortic and pulmonic stenosis is significantly increased left or right ventricular pressure with a resulting systolic pressure drop across the aortic or pulmonic valve. With severe aortic stenosis, subendocardial ischemia may result from imbalance between subendocardial oxygen demand and oxygen delivery according to concepts relating to diastolic [DPTI] and systolic [SPTI] pressure time indexes. These indexes are essentially areas between the left ventricular and aortic pressure tracings during diastole and systole. Evidence of inadequate subendocardial oxygen exists when the DPTI x arterial oxygen content/ SPTI decreases below 10. When very severe in infancy both aortic and pulmonic stenosis may cause congestive cardiac failure (2).

Natural History: Complications of aortic or pulmonic stenosis relate to severity. If mild, there is no alteration in longevity and the patient is ordinarily symptom free. In moderate to severe aortic stenosis, the risk of sudden death exists. This risk is not as significant for pulmonic stenosis. If no progression of stenosis occurs by about 6 years of age, then further significant progression is unlikely.

Physical Findings: There is seldom any alteration of growth in mild to moderate aortic or pulmonic stenosis. Even with severe degrees of stenosis, little growth problem exists unless CHF develops. Cyanosis is not present in isolated lesions. Systolic thrills are often present over the upper right sternal border with aortic stenosis and over the upper left sternal border with pulmonic stenosis. Systolic thrills in the suprasternal notch region are also quite common, especially with aortic stenosis. Generally a suprasternal notch thrill could indicate aortic or pulmonic stenosis, aortic coarctation, or PDA.

With aortic stenosis the apical impulse is usually in a normal position and becomes somewhat prominent with increasing degrees of stenosis. The first heart sound is normal; the second heart sound is more narrowly split as the degree of aortic stenosis increases. However, when the stenosis is very severe, the intensity of the aortic component of the second heart sound becomes so decreased that it may not be heard, and the child will have a single second heart sound. A systolic ejection click is present along the LV ejection path between the apex and upper right sternal border [aortic area]. It is constant and disappears only with very severe degrees of aortic stenosis. A fourth heart sound would reflect severe stenosis. The presence of hepatomegaly depends upon the presence of CHF. Pulses are normal with mild to moderate aortic stenosis but become diminished with severe stenosis.

With pulmonic stenosis, the apical impulse is usually normal. An RV lift or tap is palpable at the lower left sternal border with increasing severity. The first heart sound is normal. The second heart sound becomes more widely split with increasing severity until as in aortic stenosis when the degree of pulmonary stenosis becomes severe, the pulmonary component becomes inaudible and the second heart sound appears single. The ejection click of pulmonic stenosis is maximal over the pulmonary area at the upper left sternal border and is usually intermittent. A moderate systolic ejection murmur is present over the pulmonic or aortic area, depending upon the valve involved. With aortic stenosis, there is superior radiation of the murmur toward the neck. The murmur becomes longer with increasing degrees of stenosis in both lesions.

Differential Diagnosis: The major differential for mild degrees of pulmonic stenosis would be ASD. In the case of pulmonic stenosis, the systolic ejection murmur is usually more harsh, a systolic click is present and the second heart sound moves slightly, physiologically, although widely split. Systolic thrills would be evidence for stenosis rather than ASD. With ASD, the RV impulse is more hyperdynamic rather than forceful as it is with pulmonic stenosis.

ECG Findings: With increasing degrees of pulmonary stenosis, one most often finds increasing evidence for RVH with right axis deviation of the QRS axis as well. Right atrial abnormality is possible for very severe stenosis. With aortic stenosis, a very important notion is that the ECG may be perfectly normal in face of extreme stenosis. Often, however, if no overt LVH is present in face of severe aortic stenosis, then ST-T wave abnormalities or suggestion of LV ischemia is present.

ECHO Findings: Cross-sectional echo can be helpful in demonstration of a thickened, stenotic aortic or pulmonic valve. It may also elaborate a bicuspid aortic valve or dysplastic pulmonic valve. Doppler studies, however, are definitive in demonstration of stenotic lesions and recent data suggest that Doppler study allows very accurate non-invasive estimates of instantaneous pressure difference across aortic or pulmonic stenoses. ECHO/Doppler studies would also allow differentiation of other levels of obstruction other than classical valvar aortic stenosis, such as membranous sub-valvar stenosis or supravalvar aortic stenosis.

Radiographic Findings: Radiographic findings are usually normal with aortic stenosis apart from demonstration of dilatation of the ascending aorta. With pulmonary stenosis, one is usually able to find evidence for main pulmonary arterial enlargement. Pulmonary vascular markings are normal in both lesions.

Cardiac Cath: Cardiac catheterization is becoming more important as an interventional tool rather than a diagnostic tool. The standard pressure differences across stenotic aortic or pulmonic valves that warrant intervention have classically been from cath procedures. It is important to consider cardiac output at the time of cath and the systolic flow across the valve. Pressure drop alone can be misleading if cardiac index is very low from cardiac failure. In order to consider both the pressure drop and the flow across a stenotic valve Gorlin and Gorlin derived an hydraulic formula for estimation of aortic or pulmonary valve areas as follows: Valve area [cm^2] = [stroke volume/systolic ejection time]/ 44.5 x [P2-P1]$^{1/2}$, where P2-P1 is the area between the LV and aortic pressure curves during systole (3). Bache modified this formula to enable similar estimates of valve area without actually performing calculation of area under the LV and aortic pressure tracing curves, using peak to peak systolic pressure differences as follows: Valve area [cm^2] = [stroke volume/systolic ejection time]/ 37.8 x [PSPD+10]$^{1/2}$, where PSPD is the peak systolic pressure difference between the LV and aorta (4).

Similar Lesions Physiologically: An interesting variation of valvar aortic stenosis is subvalvar membranous aortic stenosis where a systolic ejection click is less common and associated aortic insufficiency is more common. ECHO can differentiate this level of aortic stenosis, which must be considered in any patient with stenosis of the ostium infundibulum as well. Another variation is supravalvar aortic stenosis which is quite common in children with William syndrome, who also have elfin facies, a high incidence of mental retardation, and probable infantile hypercalcemia. In this interesting variation, one notices accentuation of the aortic component of the second sound rather than a decrease, because the high pressure chamber is above the valve. With this level of aortic stenosis systolic ejection clicks are not common and aortic insufficiency is less common compared with subvalvar aortic stenosis. Systolic thrills and murmur transmission extends more superiorly than with other forms of aortic stenosis, generally. Another interesting feature is the finding of a lower left arm pressure compared with the right arm. This has been attributed to dissipation of potential energy in the right subclavian artery because of geometric relationships set up by this level of stenosis. Peripheral pulmonary stenosis is also often found in this group of patients.

Interesting variations of pulmonary stenosis include membranous stenosis of the ostium infundibulum and anomalous RV muscle bundle causing obstruction within the RV.

Management: Relief of moderate to severe degrees of aortic and pulmonary stenosis is now possible with interventional cardiac catheterization using balloon dilatation techniques. Early results are extremely encouraging and appear to have an advantage over open heart surgery regarding relief of stenosis safely. The appearance of new aortic insufficiency after the procedure is no greater than with surgery and usually less significant. With pulmonary stenosis, balloon dilatation is the therapy of choice whereas relief of aortic stenosis is still under investigation using these exciting techniques. Dysplastic pulmonary valve stenosis, which is usually familial, is usually considered unamenable to balloon dilatation although many centers will try this method before surgical relief of the stenosis. Many large centers have their own criteria to decide which degree of aortic stenosis requires relief but generally pressure drops equal to or greater than 55-65 mm Hg with a normal cardiac index would warrant relief of aortic stenosis; whereas many centers would recommend relieve of less severe pulmonary stenosis in the range of 40-50 mm Hg with normal cardiac index, because the procedure appears so safe, and avoids open heart surgery. The development of interventional cardiac cath techniques such as above, are amongst the most exciting developments in pediatric cardiology.

VII. OBSTRUCTION TO LV AND RV INFLOW PATHWAYS:

Physiology: Consequences of severe LV inflow obstruction result in significant left atrial hypertension with resulting increases in pulmonary arterial pressures and possible pulmonary edema. If there is an associated atrial septal defect, a large left to right shunt at the atrial level is usual. Etiologies of LV inflow obstruction are interesting and varied, including congenital mitral stenosis, supravalvar mitral valve fibrous stenosing ring, parachute mitral valve [one papillary muscle attachment limits mitral valve motion; this lesion may also be associated with supravalvar stenosing ring above the mitral valve, subaortic obstruction, and aortic coarctation; in this instance it is often referred to as Shone syndrome]. Other examples include many forms of Cor triatriatum anomalies where all pulmonary veins drain to a chamber that is not completely incorporated into the left atrium. There is subsequent flow from this chamber to the left atrium or to the right and then the left atrium. Flow into the left atrium is often impeded and the lesions can mimic mitral stenosis.

Consequences of severe RV inflow obstruction involve systemic venous hypertension with engorgement of the liver and impediment of venous return from the upper and lower circulations. If severe, there must be an atrial communication in order to decompress the right atrium, resulting in a marked atrial right to left shunt and bordering on a common mixing lesion at the atrial level. The major lesion associated with RV inflow obstruction is congenital tricuspid stenosis, which is very rare and often associated with severe underdevelopment or hypoplasia of the RV. If extreme, physiology is no different than that encountered with tricuspid atresia.

Natural History: Significant obstruction to either RV or LV inflow pathways must be relieved or palliative atrial septectomy must be performed. Milder forms may not have any adverse effects and actually go undetected for protracted periods.

Physical Findings: The classical finding of mitral stenosis is a diastolic rumble over the mitral area at the apex. There is presystolic accentuation, ordinarily. Fourth heart sounds may be present as well.

Findings of tricuspid stenosis are similar with a diastolic rumble over the tricuspid area at the lower left sternal border, unless the stenosis is so severe that little flow crosses the tricuspid valve.

Differential Diagnosis: The exact etiology to ventricular inflow obstruction is usually identified at cross sectional ECHO and Doppler study.

ECG Findings: No specific ECG pattern is present with inflow obstruction to a ventricle. One would certainly expect right atrial or left atrial abnormality to manifest. If significant pulmonary hypertension exists with LV inflow obstruction then one would likely appreciate evidence for RVH as well.

ECHO Findings: As noted above, ECHO is quite accurate in elaborating the exact nature of the ventricular inflow obstruction. Doppler study aids in assessing severity.

Radiographic Findings: No specific radiographic findings are present with this group of lesions but left atrial enlargement is associated with LV inflow obstruction and right atrial enlargement with RV inflow obstruction. Some papers indicate that there are specific radiographic findings related to parachute mitral valve; however, ECHO is a much more definitive way to elaborate this diagnosis.

Cardiac Cath: Because of the rare nature of this group of lesions, not much literature exists on usual cath findings. However, one would expect variable degrees of left atrial and pulmonary arterial hypertension with LV inflow obstruction and variable degrees of right atrial hypertension with RV inflow obstruction. Shunt at the atrial levels could also be estimated. Some of the lesions may become amenable to interventional cath relief by balloon dilatation, but inadequate data exist to predict this with any accuracy.

Similar Lesions Physiologically: Extremes of ventricular inflow obstruction would behave similarly to mitral or tricuspid atresia.

Management: Most forms of ventricular inflow obstruction are surgically correctable, including supravalvar mitral stenosing rings, Cor triatriatum. Depending upon circumstances, one might need to resort to corrections similar to tricuspid atresia, such as the Fontan procedure, if the tricuspid stenosis is very severe and associated with RV hypoplasia. Mitral valve replacement may be necessary for severe parachute mitral valve. This would be deferred as much as possible to avoid repeated valve replacement necessitated by growth of the child.

VIII. REGURGITANT LESIONS OF THE ATRIOVENTRICULAR VALVES:

Physiology: The most important example of this group of lesions is Ebstein anomaly of the tricuspid valve which is a spectrum of increasingly severe degrees of tricuspid insufficiency associated with diminishing function of the RV. The lesion is basically a result of abnormal development of the septal tricuspid leaflet which is adherent to RV septum for a varying length. The more length, the more severe the consequences. If very severe, the tricuspid regurgitation becomes associated with atrial right to left shunting resulting in significant cyanosis. Poor RV function leads to inadequate pulmonary blood flow.

There is a transient form of neonatal tricuspid insufficiency which can be documented by Doppler study, and likely results from an excessive increase in pulmonary vascular resistance postnatally in addition to a decrease in RV function. This form is usually not severe enough to cause CHF or other symptoms.

Mitral insufficiency is rare congenitally and in earlier years was almost always associated with acute rheumatic fever. Presently a small group of children with mitral valve prolapse manifest mitral insufficiency, which is usually mild. Severe mitral insufficiency may be associated with significant CHF and left atrial hypertension as well as LV volume overload.

Children with any endocardial cushion defect such as ostium primum ASD or complete atrioventricular canal, may have varying degrees of mitral and/or tricuspid regurgitation. Interestingly infants with Down syndrome and this group of lesions tend to have a less severe degree of atrioventricular valve regurgitation.

Natural History: Ebstein anomaly is very variable in outcome and natural history. Mild forms may go unnoticed for one or two decades whereas very severe forms may cause death in the neonatal period.

Rheumatic mitral insufficiency was usually amenable to adequate stabilization with anti-congestive medication and with anti-inflammatory agents. A small subgroup of children required emergency mitral valve replacement.

Mitral valve prolapse seldom causes symptomatic mitral insufficiency in children.

Physical Findings: Mitral insufficiency is usually associated with a hyperdynamic LV impulse and possible mild to moderate cardiomegaly. The first heart sound may be difficult to appreciate because of the early onset of the murmur, which is a long blowing systolic murmur maximal at the apex with radiation to the left axilla. The second heart sound is normal unless significant pulmonary hypertension is present, in which case the pulmonary component may be accentuated.

Significant tricuspid insufficiency results in a slightly hyperdynamic RV impulse. The first heart sound may also be difficult to appreciate because of the long blowing "superficial" systolic murmur at the lower left sternal border. At times such a murmur may mimic that of a VSD. However, the VSD murmur is more harsh and less "superficial" or less "scratchy" in quality. The second heart sound is normal with the exception of patients with Ebstein anomaly, where the second heart sound may be widely split secondary to a complete right bundle branch block.

Differential Diagnosis: Regurgitant A-V valve murmurs occasionally resemble those of VSD as noted above.

ECG Findings: Patients with Ebstein anomaly most often have either Wolff-Parkinson-White syndrome or complete right bundle branch block on the ECG. Other forms of A-V valve regurgitation are unassociated with specific findings on ECG other than expected right or left atrial abnormalities. Patients with mitral valve prolapse most often have T wave inversion or flattening in the infero-lateral leads [II,III,AVF,V5-6]. They also have a high risk of ventricular or atrial arrhythmias.

ECHO Findings: The ECHO/Doppler study is quite diagnostic of Ebstein anomaly and would also elaborate associated pulmonary stenosis. Similarly mitral valve prolapse is found on approximately 80-95% of ECHO studies, if present clinically. The severity of tricuspid or mitral insufficiency may be estimated by Doppler study as well.

Radiographic Findings: In severe forms of Ebstein anomaly one expects right atrial enlargement with significant cardiomegaly and decreased pulmonary vascular markings.

Left atrial enlargement is present with significant mitral insufficiency which may also cause CHF with its typical findings on radiographs of the chest.

Cardiac Cath: Diagnosis by cath is not essential in Ebstein anomaly because of ECHO technology, however, one should assess the possible degree of pulmonary stenosis and right to left atrial shunt by cath. Early cath studies included sophisticated simultaneous electrophysiological studies to document the presence of Ebstein anomaly. One would find right atrial pressure contours with associated evidence for tricuspid insufficiency in a chamber that one recorded RV pressures, indicating "atrialization" of the non-functioning portion of the RV.

Cath is no longer warranted for assessment of isolated mitral valve prolapse.

Management: Tricuspid valve replacement may be the only therapy available for the neonate in extremis with Ebstein anomaly. Interestingly, although the pulmonary blood flow is reduced, aortico-pulmonary shunts are not well tolerated in these patients and should not be performed as palliation, even in the presence of severe pulmonary stenosis.

Surgery is almost never required for mitral valve prolapse. Patients with acute rheumatic mitral insufficiency seldom required surgical replacement of the valve.

Therapy for cardiac arrhythmias or CHF would be no different for this group of lesions.

IX. REGURGITANT LESIONS OF THE SEMILUNAR VALVES:

Physiology: Aortic or pulmonary insufficiency results in volume overload of the respective ventricle. Aortic insufficiency may be associated with bicuspid aortic valve, high VSD in a supracristal position near the aortic valve, or in association with acute rheumatic fever.

Isolated pulmonary insufficiency is rare with the exception of unguarded pulmonary valve where no pulmonary valve structure developed. It occurs frequently following correction of tetralogy of Fallot.

Natural History: Whereas pulmonary insufficiency is ordinarily very well tolerated, patients with moderate to severe degrees of aortic insufficiency may develop irreversible left ventricular damage. Such patients obviously require surgical intervention.

Physical Findings: The semilunar valve insufficiency murmurs are decrescendo, blowing almost echoing diastolic murmurs. In the instance of aortic insufficiency, the murmur is maximal along the LV ejection path between the apex and upper right sternal border. It may even be maximal at the mid left sternal border. It occurs immediately after the aortic component of the second heart sound. With pulmonary insufficiency, the murmur is loudest between the upper left and lower left sternal border and occurs after the pulmonary component of the second heart sound.

Differential Diagnosis: Few lesions mimic the murmurs of aortic or pulmonary insufficiency. Coronary arterio-venous malformations result in long diastolic murmurs which are not truly regurgitant in quality, and are often maximal only at the mid left sternal edge.

ECG Findings: No specific ECG findings are associated with semilunar valve insufficiency. If severe the respective insufficiencies would be associated with LVH or RVH as well as possible respective atrial abnormalities.

ECHO Findings: There are now excellent ECHO/Doppler capabilities to elaborate the presence and relative severity of semilunar valve insufficiency. Absence of the pulmonary valve would also be demonstrated with ECHO.

Radiographic Findings: Dilatation of the aortic root or main pulmonary artery would be present with significant insufficiency of the aortic or pulmonic valves. LV or RV enlargement is also expected with significant degrees of insufficiency.

Cardiac Cath: The necessity for cardiac cath is limited now with the development of non-invasive ECHO/Doppler technique. Nevertheless, cineangiography remains useful for qualitative analysis of the insufficiency.

Management: Aortic valve replacement is necessary for degrees of aortic insufficiency likely to result in irreversible damage to the LV.

Pulmonary valve replacement is almost never necessary, and it is generally believed that pulmonary insufficiency is quite well tolerated. Patients with unguarded pulmonary valve eventually require pulmonary valve replacement.

X. MISCELLANEOUS LESIONS INCLUDING PDA DEPENDENT LESIONS AND CORONARY ARTERIAL MALFORMATIONS :

Aortic Coarctation: Aortic coarctation is an interesting lesion that often manifests in the neonatal period. Importantly it is a very dynamic lesion in the immediate newborn period because of a possible associated patent ductus arteriosus [PDA]. Even if severe, aortic coarctation may not manifest until spontaneous closure of a PDA occurs [see Fig. 6.8]. Once faced with such a sudden, marked increase in afterload, the neonatal heart often develops CHF. Diagnosis of aortic coarctation is easy with appreciation of diminished or absent femoral pulses in face of normal or increased upper extremity pulses. With severe CHF, however, all pulses may appear diminished.

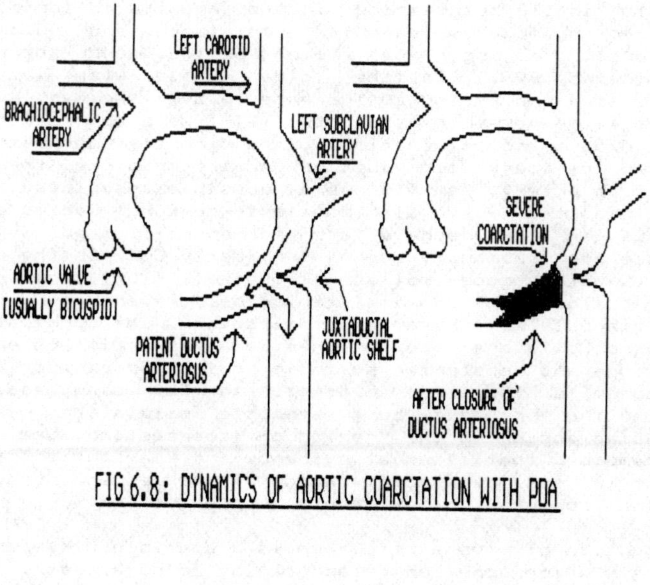

FIG 6.8: DYNAMICS OF AORTIC COARCTATION WITH PDA

In the newborn manifesting CHF in association with aortic coarctation, Prostaglandin E1 infusion may be life-saving, until surgical intervention is possible. Other cardiac findings in the neonate include an RV heave at the lower left sternal border as well as a narrowly split second heart sound with an increased pulmonary component. The pulmonary hypertension develops in the neonate develops from an increase in LV afterload resulting in an increased pulmonary vascular resistance. With CHF, a prominent third heart sound is often present. A fourth heart sound may also develop, reflecting difficult filling of the LV by the left atrium. Sixty percent of patients with aortic coarctation have an associated bicuspid aortic valve, in which case one appreciates a systolic click upon exam as well. Other physical findings are not specific and include a non-specific short, harsh systolic ejection murmur anywhere over the precordium or over the aortic area as well as over the posterior left hemithorax.

ECG with aortic coarctation in the neonate reflects the increased pulmonary vascular resistance and pulmonary hypertension during that time period, and therefore demonstrates RVH. In the older child with systemic hypertension and prolonged increase in LV afterload, LVH is present with possible associated ST-T wave abnormalities. Echocardiographic examination often directly demonstrates the area of coarctation just beyond the origin of the left subclavian artery as well as a possible associated PDA. Bicuspid aortic valve also manifests on ECHO. Radiographic findings in the neonate are non-specific and involve evidence for pulmonary edema from early CHF. In the older patient with good collateral vessel flow, one notes notching along the proximal third of the anterior ribs, from internal mammary artery dilatation. The correlate of increased collateral flow on physical exam is interscapular pulsations and posterior systolic bruits. On barium filled esophagram in the older patient, an "E" sign appears, representing pre and post stenotic dilatation of the descending aorta in the region of coarctation. One must also remember that if usual evidence for coarctation is not present in the juxtaductal region of the descending aorta, abdominal coarctation may rarely be present.

Interruption of the aortic arch is a possible differential diagnosis which one can elaborate by cardiac cath. With interruption of the aortic arch, one is also able to note a decreased descending aortic oxygen saturation [umbilical artery sample], compared with a normal or at least a higher ascending aortic oxygen saturation [right radial artery sample]. This lesion must be associated with a widely patent ductus arteriosus to supply descending aortic flow. prostaglandin E1 infusion is critical in infants with this lesion, once the PDA begins to close. Whereas interruption of the aortic arch requires immediate surgery, many children with coarctation tolerate the lesion well and come to surgery as late as 4-6 years of age. Some are not detected until much later because some physicians do not routinely palpate all four extremity pulses.

Therapy involves surgical resection of the coarctation using a subclavian flap technique or direct end to end anastomosis. Balloon dilatation of native coarctation is now associated with a small incidence of late, serious aneurysms of the aorta. Significant mortality has also been reported for balloon dilatation of recurrent aortic coarctation, for which reason this technique should be limited to research centers only, until more data are available. One group reported a significant prolongation of the QTc interval during the first 1-4 hours after balloon dilatation of aortic coarctation. This would have the potential for serious ventricular arrhythmias, theoretically (5). Possible refinement in balloon dilatation techniques may again allow these to become the therapy of choice in the future. A fascinating observation using these techniques is the absence of rebound systemic hypertension, so often following surgical correction. Additionally, balloon dilatation techniques have not thus far been associated with post-coarctectomy syndrome, which involves extreme abdominal pain from mesenteric arteritis. To avoid this common postoperative complication, surgeons usually continue the patient's NPO status several days after surgery with mild NG suctioning as well. Systemic hypertension after relief of aortic coarctation may be so severe as to warrant stabilization with intravenous nitroprusside [0.5-1.5 mcg/kg/min as a continuous drip]. Interestingly old fashioned therapy with combination reserpine [0.07 mg/kg/dose IM every 12-24 hours] and hydralazine [0.15 mg/kg/dose IV slowly over 30 minutes every 4-6 hours], also works extremely well. Once stable, if long term therapy of systemic hypertension is necessary, these children usually respond to propranolol 1-4 mg/kg/day divided into every 6 or 12 hour doses.

PDA dependent lesions: Lesions that must be associated with patent ductus arteriosus for newborn survival include pulmonary atresia and hypoplastic left heart syndrome. In the instance of pulmonary atresia it should be apparent that survival depends upon delivery of pulmonary blood flow to the lungs by a PDA because of an absent pulmonary valve. Early stabilization requires prostaglandin E1, prior to early palliative shunt procedures. Diagnosis by ECHO is possible, but cardiac catheterization is necessary to elaborate the pulmonary arterial vessel supply and configuration in order to plan future correction or palliation.

In the case of hypoplastic left heart syndrome the infant must have a PDA to sustain the systemic circulation in face of aortic atresia. Additionally, an atrial communication is necessary especially with associated mitral atresia. VSD is quite common, also. This particular lesion is involved with extreme controversy. It usually presents early, when the PDA begins to close, resulting in circulatory collapse. Fig. 6.9 demonstrates the basic circulation in an infant

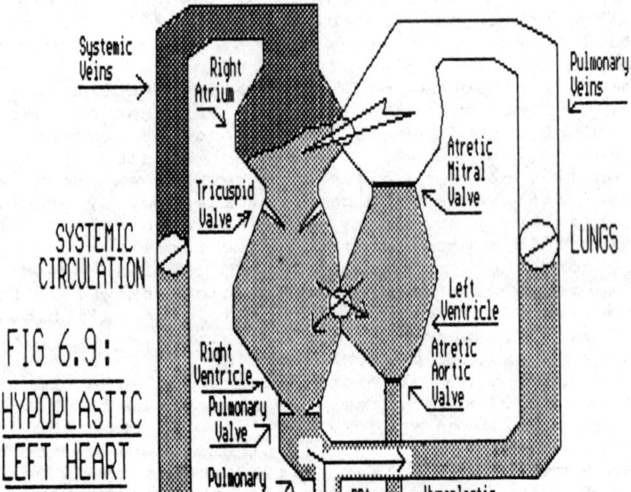

FIG 6.9: HYPOPLASTIC LEFT HEART SYNDROME

with hypoplastic left heart syndrome including aortic and mitral atresia with atrial septal defect. The infant appears gray from poor systemic perfusion and manifests grunting with other signs of CHF. Diagnosis may be extremely difficult in the infant with large PDA, because of the resulting stabilization of systemic flow. However, at a minimum, the physician should be able to appreciate a single second heart sound with no functional aortic valve present, after the immediate newborn period. ECHO study enables definitive diagnosis. ECG usually demonstrates decreased leftward forces [i.e., decreased R waves in leads V5-6]. Corrective procedures are available but often involve prolonged maintenance on ventilatory support and eventual death. Many believe that no intervention should take place in face of these results. However, logically, surgery should continue at a few select centers with experience with these lesions until more data are available pertaining to long term survival and quality of life. Importantly, early data suggested little or no significant associated malformations in infants with hypoplastic left heart syndrome. This was a major impetus to develop procedures to help these infants. Recent data suggests that a subgroup of these infants do have other malformations, some of which involve central nervous system defects such as absence of the corpus callosum. One could question heroic measures in this subgroup.

Anomalous origin of the left coronary artery: It is important to recognize the possibility of anomalous origin of the left coronary artery from the pulmonary artery because it is now correctable surgically. This lesion manifests in overt antero-lateral myocardial infarction once the high newborn pulmonary vascular resistance decreases and the coronary circulation cannot be sustained from the low pressure pulmonary artery. These infants are classically irritable and unconsolable. The ECG demonstrates changes consistent with antero-lateral myocardial infarction which is otherwise extraordinarily rare in the pediatric patient.

Some children recover from the early myocardial infarction and develop diastolic murmurs of retrograde flow from the coronary arteries to the pulmonary arteries. Their ECG still manifest classical signs of old antero-lateral myocardial infarction with prominent "Q" waves in leads I,AVL, V5-6. Surgical correction with reimplantation of the anomalous coronary into the aortic root is still necessary.

Notes

1. Stanger P. Cardiac Malpositions. In Rudolph AM [ed], Hoffman JIE [coed]: *Pediatrics*, 7th Edition. Norwalk, Appleton-Century-Crofts, 1982, p 1240.

2. Lewis AL, Heymann MA, Stanger P, Hoffman JIE, Rudolph AM: Evaluation of subendocardial ischemia in valvar aortic stenosis in children. *Circulation* 49:978, 1975.

3. Gorlin R, Gorlin SG: Hydraulic formula for calculation of area of stenotic mitral valve, other cardiac valves, and central circulatory shunts. *Am Heart J* 41:1, 1951.

4. Bache RJ, Jorgensen CR, Wang Y: Simplified estimate of aortic valve area. *Brit Heart J* 34:408, 1972.

5. Stanger P: Personal communication, September, 1986.

Chapter 7

Pediatric Cardiac Emergencies

CONGESTIVE CARDIAC FAILURE (1)

Congestive heart failure (CHF) may be defined as the inability of the heart to meet a patient's circulatory needs. Although clinical findings of congestive cardiac failure are usually apparent to the physician caring for pediatric patients, the presentation of an infant or child in congestive heart failure may be subtle. Therapeutic intervention is an emergency in either event.

Etiology and onset: Congestive cardiac failure in infants and children generally results either from volume or pressure overload, or from intrinsic myocardial dysfunction associated with cardiomyopathy, myocarditis, metabolic derangement (e.g., severe hypoglycemia or hypocalcemia), or cardiac arrhythmias. Whereas obstructive lesions such as severe valvar aortic stenosis or aortic coarctation may present shortly after birth,"dependent" shunt lesions which allow a progressive increase in pulmonary blood flow only after the high neonatal pulmonary vascular resistance decreases, usually do not cause overt CHF until four to eight weeks of age. Also contributing to difficulty at this time is the physiological anemia which may interfere with adequate systemic oxygen transport. Antero-lateral myocardial infarction associated with rare aberrant left coronary arterial origin from the main pulmonary artery, may also cause CHF, once the high neonatal pulmonary vascular resistance decreases. Interestingly, although often viewed as a fixed obstruction, aortic coarctation is potentially a dynamic lesion in the neonatal period, not manifesting until closure of a patent ductus arteriosus. It is not uncommon for a newborn to be discharged from the nursery with adequate femoral pulses, only to return several weeks later in severe congestive heart failure with absent femoral pulses. Lesions which may also present with CHF in the immediate newborn period include cardiomyopathy, myocarditis, paroxysmal supraventricular tachycardia, and rarely, congenital cerebral arterio-venous malformations (Vein of Galen Aneurysm). The latter lesion is an example of an "obligatory" shunt from a high to low pressure system. Such a shunt develops regardless of the pulmonary to systemic vascular resistance ratios.

Patient history: Parents of children manifesting CHF are often the first to notice a significant change in the child's behavior. Too often physicians overlook the parents' concern about easy tiring with feeding, poor weight gain, dry cough, and irritability, which are all associated with CHF. The typical infant or child in CHF tires easily during feeding, often in association with increased respiratory rate and effort. Occasionally there is a history of frequent regurgitation. End expiratory "grunting", intercostal, subcostal, suprasternal retractions, and flaring of the ala nasae are often noticed by the parents and reflect the respiratory complications of pulmonary edema. "Grunting" appears to reflect the infant's need to increase end-expiratory pressure to keep terminal alveoli open in face of pulmonary edema. With continued stress, endogenous catecholamine secretion results in easy diaphoresis, especially during periods of activity such as feeding. The very young infant is unable to display diaphoresis, however. Mottling of the extremities, pallor, a gray hue, or mild cyanosis are late manifestations of CHF in the infant and young child. Some very observant parents or grand-parents are able to notice an excessive precordial impulse in the infant with shunt volume overload when they place the infant over their shoulder for comforting.

General Physical Findings: Because the newborn's myocardium is unable to increase stroke volume, the only way to increase cardiac output is to increase heart rate. Although tachycardia, tachypnea, and cardiomegaly are the basic findings in any infant suffering from CHF, there are other important aspects of the physical examination. On inspection, one usually observes an irritable, fretful, pallid, dusky or slightly cyanotic infant in significant respiratory distress, manifested by tachypnea, thoracic retractions, flaring of the ala nasae, and "grunting." With crying, the infant soon becomes diaphoretic and more dyspneic. Subtle edema of the dorsa of the hands and feet represents dependent edema based upon the usual recumbent position of the infant. Precordial palpation may demonstrate marked cardiac hyperactivity with a hyperdynamic apical impulse displaced one to two centimeters left of the midclavicular line. With an obstructive lesion, a thrusting, prominent precordial impulse may be present. Hepatomegaly is usually marked with a dull liver edge palpable three to five centimeters below the right costal margin. Peripheral pulses are usually decreased in late stages of CHF. The lungs may be clear to auscultation, but occasionally one appreciates slight wheezing or basal rales. The latter findings occur much less commonly in the pediatric patient compared with the adult. On auscultation of the heart, the physician usually has a sense that something is abnormal. Even if cardiac murmurs are absent or non-specific, the heart sounds appear pathological. The first and/or second heart sounds may be indistinct; the second heart sound may appear single or narrowly split with a loud pulmonary component; a prominent third and/or fourth heart sound may give a classical gallop rhythm; a prominent systolic click may be present.

Initial Stabilization: Place the infant or child in a semi-upright position with the head elevated to between 25 and 35 degrees. Carefully control temperature with a radiant warmer in the young infant. If dusky or overtly cyanotic, give the patient oxygen. An FiO_2 of .3 to .5 is usually adequate and, in fact, higher concentrations may acutely decrease pulmonary vascular resistance, thereby increasing pulmonary blood flow in "dependent" shunts associated with defects such as ventricular septal defect, patent ductus arteriosus, or complete A-V canal. Intravenous access is indicated in all initial stages of management because of poor peripheral perfusion and to provide access if emergency drugs become necessary. One may start with low maintenance fluids (80-100 ml/kg/day or 800-1200 ml/square meter/day), using 5% glucose water, 0.2 normal saline and added maintenance KCl (2-3 mEq/kg/day:only after urine flow or adequate renal function is established). EXTREME CARE IS NECESSARY FOR ALL IV LINES REGARDING AIR, BECAUSE LESIONS ASSOCIATED WITH ANATOMICAL RIGHT TO LEFT SHUNTS PERMIT SYSTEMIC AIR EMBOLIZATION.

To provide sedation and because of its effect in relieving pulmonary edema, give morphine sulfate (0.05-0.2 mg/Kg, intravenously). At the higher doses, care must be taken not to depress ventilation.

Even prior to digitalization, give a fast acting diuretic as soon as possible. Furosemide, 0.5 to 1.0 mg/kg intravenously, results in a prompt diuresis. In the unusual event that furosemide is ineffective, ethacrynic acid (1.0 mg/kg IV only) may be tried. Correct metabolic acidemia as soon as possible to improve myocardial function. In mild, chronic CHF, arterial blood gas analysis usually demonstrates balanced metabolic alkalosis secondary to hyperventilation resulting in hypocarbia. In severe or late stage CHF, carbon dioxide retention and significant metabolic acidosis are often present.

Baseline laboratory and non-invasive findings (NOTE: PROVIDE INITIAL STABILIZATION BEFORE ORDERING LENGTHY STUDIES OR LABORATORY DATA):

Echocardiography is one of the most useful non-invasive tools in assessing major intracardiac defects. Poor myocardial contractility is also reflected in two-dimensional and M-mode echocardiograms.

Electrocardiography is essential to elaborate cardiac arrhythmias. In other etiologies, an ECG is of little help in clarifying the diagnosis of CHF, other than pointing to congenital or acquired cardiac abnormalities. A baseline ECG is necessary prior to digitalization, however.

Radiographs of the chest demonstrate significant cardiomegaly. Rare exceptions include lesions that impede pulmonary venous return to the heart such as obstructed total anomalous venous return below the diaphragm or Cor Triatriatum. Pulmonary venous engorgement, with or without increased pulmonary vascular markings, is most often present. Specific cardiac silhouette configurations may aid in the diagnosis of underlying congenital heart disease, but Echocardiography is much more specific.

Hemoglobin and hematocrit determination is useful for possible further management, in that physiological anemia may be the cause of worsening CHF. Significant anemia may require slow packed RBC transfusion. Polycythemia reflects significant systemic desaturation.

Serum BUN and creatinine may be increased, reflecting pre-renal failure as well as poor fluid intake.
Serum potassium is ordinarily normal but should be documented before the second digitalizing dose of digoxin.
Baseline serum Na and Cl should also be determined.
Determination of Serum glucose and calcium are important because hypoglycemia or hypocalcemia may be associated with CHF in the young child. Correct hypocalcemia before using digitalis, if possible. (See caution below.)

Arterial blood gas data (usually right radial) are necessary to quantitate the degree of hypoxemia and/or metabolic acidemia.

Digitalization: While the above measures usually improve the infant's clinical condition significantly, digitalis remains one of the most essential drugs to treat CHF. Although several forms of Digitalis are available, most Pediatric Cardiologists prefer Digoxin, largely because the much shorter half-life compared with Digitoxin, allows safe, rapid re-adjustment of doses. Recent studies in animal models have demonstrated that digitalis appears to alter or improve myocardial performance to a lesser degree in the young myocardium compared with the adult myocardium. Whereas digitalis was often "pushed" to toxicity in the past, there appears to be no rationale for using very high doses in infants and children. Recent dose range recommendations reflect this.

Although the approach to digitalization varies slightly in different centers, basically, one administers a total digitalizing dose (TDD) in three (3) divided doses over 8 to 16 hours. Twelve (12) hours later, place the pediatric patient on a Total Daily Maintenance (TMD) of digoxin, divided into two (2) doses/day (i.e., given q 12 h). The division of the Total Daily Maintenance Dose into two doses allows for accidental administration of two doses given close together by different family members. In that event, one needs only to skip one of the daily maintenance doses. Unfortunately this happens frequently.

Route of Administration: Initial digitalization should be done INTRAVENOUSLY, to assure proper levels of digoxin. There is no place for intramuscular digitalization because of poor peripheral perfusion associated with CHF and because it is now well known that this route is associated with extreme pain. Only rarely is oral digitalization acceptable. INTRAVENOUS DIGITALIZATION REQUIRES EXTREME CARE IN CALCULATION OF DOSAGE AND IN ADMINISTRATION. One center reported several instances of serious digitalis toxicity in premature infants secondary to emptying a tuberculin syringe hub dead space, when giving IV doses. After complete digitalization, it is often possible to change from an IV to an ORAL route for maintenance therapy.

Digitalization Orders and Concepts: Table 7.1 below lists recommended Total Digitalizing Doses (TDD) for different age groups. After deciding upon a TDD, order the first Digitalizing Dose at once. A convenient division of TDD is

1/3, 1/3, 1/3, spaced four to eight (4-8) hours apart. Because Digoxin Elixir bio-availability is 70-85%, compared with 100% bio-availability of the parenteral form, if one changes from IV to Oral therapy, 4/3 of the IV dose must be used orally. Conversely, 3/4 of an oral dose would be used intravenously. In older children, a new oral preparation is available (Lanoxicaps 50, 100, or 200 mcg/capsule), which has 90-100% bio-availability and therefore requires no adjustment of dosage between IV or Oral routes of administration. Because of long experience and bio-availability studies, Lanoxin (digoxin) by Burroughs-Wellcome, should be used exclusively in children, and orders should reflect this. For intravenous Lanoxin extreme care by pharmacy and by nursing is necessary to avoid using Adult Injectable Lanoxin (250 mcg/ml) instead of Pediatric Injectable (100 mcg/ml). Unfortunately vials are quite similar.

Do not write any open-ended orders for digitalization [e.g., give 10 micrograms (0.1 ml) Pediatric Lanoxin Injectable (100 mcg/ml) now and q 8 h for two more doses]. Rather, hold each Digitalization dose, after the first, until complete patient and ECG re-evaluation by the physician. If toxicity manifests after the second or third Digitalization dose, consider the total amount administered prior to that dose, the TDD for that patient and base the maintenance dose upon that amount.

Digitalization should proceed very cautiously if hypokalemia (<3.5 mEq/L) is present, thus potentiating digoxin effect. Correct hypokalemia as soon as possible, but avoid high concentrations (>20-40 mEq/L) if possible. Administer potassium only through controlled rate IV units, not by free flowing IV drip.

Once a patient is Digitalized, IV CALCIUM SHOULD NEVER BE ADMINISTERED BY BOLUS. This acutely potentiates digoxin and may result in ventricular standstill.

Recent data indicate that the lower dose ranges in the table below result in serum digoxin levels of 1.1-1.7 ng/ml, which appears to be a safe and therapeutic pediatric range (2). However, one must also consider the possible effect of endogenous digoxin-like substances on immunoassay, falsely increasing serum values.

Table 7.1: TOTAL DIGITALIZING (TDD) AND TOTAL DAILY MAINTENANCE (TMD) DOSES OF INTRAVENOUS PEDIATRIC INJECTABLE (100 mcg/ml) & PEDIATRIC LANOXIN ELIXIR (50 mcg/ml)

AGE	IV TDD (mcg/Kg)	PO TDD (mcg/Kg)	IV TMD (mcg/Kg)	PO TMD (mcg/Kg)
PREMATURE [<1 month]	15-25	20-30	20-30% OF IV TDD	20-30% OF PO TDD OR 20-30% OF IV TDD x 4/3
FULL TERM	20-30	25-35	25-35% OF IV TDD	25-35% OF PO TDD OR 20-30% OF IV TDD x 4/3
1 MO- 1 YR,12 MOS	30-50	35-60	AS ABOVE	AS ABOVE
2 YR- 4 YR,12 MOS	25-35	30-40	AS ABOVE	AS ABOVE
5 YR- 9 YRS,12 MOS	15-30	20-35	AS ABOVE	AS ABOVE
10 YRS- ADULT	08-12 (Total Max. 600-1000 mcg)	10-15 (Total Max. 750-1250 mcg)	AS ABOVE	AS ABOVE

[1] Divide TDD into Three (3) Doses such as 1/3, 1/3, 1/3 or 1/2, 1/4, 1/4

[2] Divide TMD into Two (2) Doses: 1/2, 1/2 and begin twelve (12) hours after last Digitalizing dose

[3] Based upon ventricular response rate in patients with atrial fibrillation, inotropic and ECG effects, onset of Digoxin Effect is 5-30 minutes for IV route and 0.5-2 hours for oral route. PEAK EFFECT usually occurs 1-4 hours for IV route and 2-6 hours for PO route.

[4] Any cardiac rhythm disturbance may reflect digitalis toxicity. Sinus bradycardia, conduction block, atrial tachycardia with or without A-V block, or junctional tachycardia are most common in children. Ventricular arrhythmias are less common.

[5] Anorexia, nausea, vomiting and diarrhea may occur with toxicity but are not common.

[6] Headache, weakness, apathy and visual disturbances are uncommon in children. Gynecomastia is rare (but may be associated with spironolactone).

[7] Although renal function is usually adequate in children, adjustment of the above dose recommendations is necessary in patients with renal dysfunction.

Chronic Diuretics: After initial IV Furosemide [Lasix:0.5-1.0 mg/Kg], several repeat IV doses may be necessary every 4 to 12 hours. After further stabilization of CHF, a less potent diuretic such as chlorothiazide [Diuril:50 mg/ml Suspension] may be substituted in doses of 10-20 mg/kg/dose PO every 12 hours.

If Furosemide is still necessary, an oral suspension [10 mg/ml] may be used in doses of 1-2 mg/Kg/dose every 12 hours.

Because oral potassium supplementation is usually not well tolerated, and because hyperaldosteronism has been documented in infants and children during CHF, spironolactone (Aldactone) is often added to the diuretic regimen, thus sparing potassium, and ameliorating effects of hyperaldosteronism. Total doses of Aldactone range between 2.2-2.5 mg/Kg/day divided into three daily doses [given q 8 h, in a suspension (1 mg/ml)]. There is evidence of tumor formation in rats given high doses of Aldactone and parents should been informed of this. Generally, malignant tumors occurred only at 75 times the usual human doses. If Aldactone is not used, diuretic therapy should be tried for 5 out of 7 days per week to allow renal adjustment of potassium. In addition high potassium foods should be encouraged. This would not be done if the patient was taking Aldactone.

Afterload Reduction: Although theoretically beneficial, agents such as Prazosin (Minipress) and Hydralazine (Apresoline) have been associated with mixed results in children with CHF. Because Hydralazine may also reduce pulmonary vascular resistance variably, it may in fact have deleterious effects in children with CHF because of the resulting increase in pulmonary blood flow in "dependent" lesions. In critically ill or in post-operative cardiac patients, short acting nitroprusside [0.5-1.5 mcg/Kg/min as continuous IV drip] may be beneficial in early management. Only a limited number of pediatric patients benefit from chronic use of Prazosin or Hydralazine. In patients with poorly controlled CHF after maximum, standard anti-congestive medication (Lanoxin/Diuretic/Aldactone), surgical intervention is necessary if feasible.

The new generation Angiotensin I-converting enzyme inhibitors such as Captopril [0.3 mg/Kg dose every 8 hours with maximum dose of 6 mg/Kg/dose], may have beneficial effects in infants and children with CHF especially in association with cardiomyopathy, but data to support this are not yet completely available.

Successful post-operative use of the intraaortic balloon has been reported in a limited number of pediatric patients, and may be used more frequently in the future.

<u>Miscellaneous</u>: Significant anemia in the young child (Hb < 11-13 G% or HCT < 35-40%), may require slow packed red blood cell transfusion. For mild anemia, iron supplement is necessary. Caloric supplementation of formula to approximately 24 cal/oz is often necessary and may be achieved with glucose polymers (Polycose) and/or medium chain triglyceride oil (MCT oil). Various 24 Cal/oz infant formulas are also available. In mild CHF not requiring diuretic therapy, low sodium infant formula such as SMA (Wyeth) may be beneficial. It is unlikely that low sodium formula is necessary in patients receiving diuretic therapy, however.

Catecholamines such as Dopamine or Epinephrine are rarely needed, except post-operatively. Prostaglandin E1 administration may be vital to stabilize the neonate with severe juxtaductal aortic coarctation (see section on the cyanotic newborn). Temporary transvenous pacing may be necessary in the neonate or older child with complete heart block. If the child requires mechanical ventilation, an end-expiratory pressure of at least 4 to 6 Torr, should be provided.

SUMMARY: Management of CHF in Infants and Children includes

1) Positioning with head elevated 25-30 degrees
2) Establishment of IV access
3) Morphine Sulfate
4) Immediate & often long term diuretic therapy
5) Digitalization
6) Use of chronic Spironolactone with other diuretics in moderate to severe CHF
7) Temporary increase in FiO2 (.3 to .5) if patient is hypoxic
8) Attention to anemia, metabolic acidemia, hypoglycemia, and hypocalcemia (CAUTION)

9) Trial on afterload reduction if CHF is not well controlled with the above measures; catecholamine infusion is rarely necessary.

10) Caloric supplementation of formula

11) Low sodium formula if diuretics are not necessary

12) In the critically ill child, catecholamines, mechanical ventilation, prostaglandin E1, temporary pacing, or emergency surgery may become necessary.

THE CYANOTIC NEWBORN, WITH EMPHASIS ON "PDA DEPENDENT LESIONS" (3)

Differentiating major etiologies of cyanosis and initial management: One of the most common pediatric emergencies is the presentation of a cyanotic newborn. Because cyanotic congenital heart disease presenting so early is often very labile, dynamic, and potentially lethal, early diagnosis and intervention are essential. The first task is differentiating pulmonary from cardiac etiologies for cyanosis in the newborn. It is generally accepted that five to ten minute administration of 100% oxygen through an efficient delivery system results in greater than a 15-20 Torr increase in right radial arterial oxygen tension, compared with room air values, in the neonate with pulmonary disease. Unfortunately a 15-20 Torr increase in right radial oxygen tension may not occur in the newborn with extreme pulmonary disease or persistent pulmonary hypertension (persistent fetal circulation). Conversely, serious cyanotic congenital cardiac defects such as Truncus Arteriosus or Total Anomalous Pulmonary Venous Return, may be associated with a significant increase in arterial oxygen tension with an FIO2 of 1.0. Hypercarbia is more often associated with pulmonary disease as are overt signs of respiratory embarrassment.

To further differentiate between pulmonary disease, persistent pulmonary hypertension (PPH), or cyanotic congenital heart disease, history and other non-invasive diagnostic tests may be helpful. The neonate product of a delivery complicated by meconium aspiration and additionally associated with hypoglycemia, hypocalcemia, and/or polycythemia is at high risk for PPH, as is the infant of a diabetic gestation. Infants of a diabetic gestation are also at high risk for congenital heart defects. High resolution two-dimensional echocardiography is ordinarily accurate in elaborating normal versus abnormal intracardiac and great vessel anatomy, as well as pulmonary venous drainage, inferior vena caval drainage, and aortic arch anatomy. Radiographs of the chest may also distinguish between a pulmonary or cardiac etiology for cyanosis, but are less specific than echocardiography.

If no immediate etiology for cyanosis becomes apparent, stabilize the neonate by correcting any metabolic acidemia and effectively providing an FiO_2 between .6 and 1.0 (endotracheal intubation and mechanical ventilation are often necessary). Arrangements for immediate transport to a tertiary intensive care nursery should be instituted at once.

PDA Dependent Lesions (Cyanotic and Acyanotic): Common cardiac etiologies for neonatal cyanosis include Complete (D-) Transposition of the Great Vessels, severe Pulmonary Stenosis or Atresia with VSD, Aortic or Pulmonary Atresia with intact ventricular septum, Tricuspid Atresia, and Total Anomalous Pulmonary Venous Return. Several of the above lesions may be categorized as patent ductus arteriosus (PDA) dependent, meaning that extra-uterine survival would be possible only with the additional existence of a PDA. Examples of such lesions include Pulmonary and Aortic Atresia, where the only access to the pulmonary or systemic circulation would be via a PDA. Other dynamic neonatal congenital cardiac complexes that would benefit by the presence of a PDA require elaboration. The first example is D-Transposition of the Great Vessels with a restrictive atrial communication and intact ventricular septum. In this instance, presence of a PDA would be the only source of admixture between pulmonary and systemic circulations. The second and third lesions are severe aortic coarctation and aortic arch interruption, which are not cyanotic lesions but share a dependency upon a PDA for initial stability. Aortic coarctation is very dynamic in the immediate newborn period, in relation to patency or closure of the ductus arteriosus. With a PDA widely open, the consequences of the usual juxtaductal shelf associated with coarctation are ameliorated and essentially not manifested. Once the PDA closes, the juxtaductal shelf becomes "pinched off" and presents the neonatal left ventricle with a sudden increase in systemic vascular resistance. With aortic arch interruption, descending aortic blood flow relates directly to the patency of a ductus arteriosus.

Use of Prostaglandin E1: The reason for emphasizing PDA dependent lesions (cyanotic and acyanotic) is that Prostaglandin E1 (Upjohn Prostin VR or alprostadil) is now available to maintain patency of the neonatal ductus arteriosus. Its proper use may result in critical, life saving intervention. Although controversial, there are those who would argue that Community Hospitals with available pediatricians, should stock Prostin VR. Conceptually, if cyanotic congenital heart disease is strongly suspected and an infant suddenly becomes unstable, administration of 0.1 mcg/Kg/min of Prostin VR by peripheral IV infusion or infusion through an umbilical arterial line, may be the only intervention that might stabilize the infant. If an increase in arterial oxygen tension and/or pH occurs, the infusion should be readjusted to the slowest, effective rate by slow decreases, usually to between .01 and .075 mcg/Kg/min. If initial response is inadequate, the infusion could be slowly increased to 0.4 mcg/Kg/min, with constant monitoring and intubation equipment available for possible apnea. If higher infusion rates fail to improve the infant's condition, the Prostin VR should be stopped, especially if persistent pulmonary hypertension is another strong possibility. Refer to the current PDR for other important considerations relating to the use of Prostin VR. Many Community Hospitals would prefer to transport the cyanotic infant after stabilization, without the use of Prostin VR. Obviously this is an individual matter.

Summary:

(1) The major task in management of the cyanotic neonate is to differentiate between severe pulmonary disease, cyanotic congenital heart disease, and persistent pulmonary hypertension (persistent fetal circulation).
(2) Transport to a tertiary intensive care nursery is almost always necessary.
(3) If the etiology to cyanosis is likely cyanotic congenital heart disease, Prostin VR (Prostaglandin E1) prior to or during transport, may be life saving.
(4) Stabilization of metabolic acidemia with sodium bicarbonate (0.5 mEq/ml in the neonate) is important.
(5) Effective delivery of an FiO_2 as high as 1.0 using mechanical ventilation, may be necessary.

HYPERCYANOTIC SPELLS (4)

Introduction: With major advances in early diagnosis, stabilization, and surgery in infants with serious congenital heart disease, it has become rare for physicians to observe serious hypercyanotic spells. Nevertheless, recognition of such an event is essential to rapid, proper therapy in this small group of infants and children.

Although such "spells" were originally described in patients with tetralogy of Fallot and thus often termed "Tet Spells", hypercyanotic spells may occur in any complex of cyanotic heart defects that includes a large ventricular septal defect (VSD) and severe pulmonary stenosis (PS). Importantly, the combination of VSD and PS results in the other markers of tetralogy of Fallot: right ventricular hypertrophy and overriding aorta (aortic dextroposition). Examples of other lesions that may allow a patient to present with hypercyanotic spells include: (1) complete A-V canal with severe PS, (2) corrected (L) transposition with large VSD and severe PS, (3) double outlet right ventricle with PS, (4) single ventricle with PS, tricuspid atresia with severe PS.

Presentation: One of the most striking aspects of hypercyanotic spells (HS) is tachypnea and hyperpnea. In fact many sources refer to these episodes as paroxysmal hyperpnea or dyspnea. The initial HS may occur as early as two to six months of age. Generally the spell occurs in association with prolonged crying and often presents upon waking in the morning. A mild spell may involve only transient pallor and hyperpnea. A serious spell involves an acute, profound increase in cyanosis, hyperpnea and agitation. If sustained, this may progress to syncope, and rarely to death.

Physiology: Without discussing theories relating to the etiology of hypercyanotic spells, it is important to present the basic physiological balance in patients with VSD and PS. An understanding of this balance leads to rational therapeutic intervention. The degree of systemic desaturation in patients with VSD and PS relates directly to the total pulmonary blood flow over a period of time. A significant decrease in pulmonary blood flow results in a decrease in highly saturated pulmonary venous return available for systemic oxygen transport. If sustained, systemic hypoxemia increases and metabolic acidemia may soon develop.

In the presence of a large VSD, right ventricular systolic pressure will equal systolic pressures in the left ventricle and aorta. The degree of right ventricular obstruction is severe and importantly may be fixed or variable (dynamic), depending upon whether the dominant obstruction is valvar, supravalvar (fixed), or infundibular (variable or dynamic). Thus, given the option of ejecting across the RV outflow or across the VSD to the aorta, the RV will eject the largest proportion of its stroke volume along the pathway of least impedance or resistance. The greater the systemic impedance, the less desirable it would be for the RV to eject along that pathway into the aorta. Conversely, if there was a sudden increase in RV outflow impedance because of more vigorous infundibular contraction, it would be more desirable for the RV to eject into the aorta, rather than into the pulmonary arteries. This delicate balance in infants and children with VSD and PS is operative constantly.

Therapy: Understanding the above physiology should allow a more rational approach to therapeutic intervention relative to a hypercyanotic spell. Initial therapy involves:

(1) Intermittent knee-chest positioning (this can be accomplished by placing the infant in a supine position facing away from you and gently bringing the knees toward the chest, after grasping behind the knees). This maneuver provides a sudden increase in systemic impedance and should be taught to all parents whose children have the potential for a hypercyanotic spell.
(2) 100% oxygen administration. This initially provides a minimal increase in systemic oxygen transport by increasing dissolved oxygen, but becomes more important as pulmonary blood flow increases, as the spell is reversed.
(3) Morphine sulfate administration (0.1-0.2 mg/Kg stat IV or SC). This intervention essentially provides enough sedation to reverse the hyperpnea which is an inefficient and deleterious breathing pattern. Morphine likely exerts other physiological effects that are helpful in aleviating a hypercyanotic spell, but these are unknown.

The above three initial phases of therapy should be outlined in detail for parents, so that intervention may be started during transport to the hospital. If the above measures are inadequate in stabilizing the infant, it is likely that the spell was so severe and sustained as to cause metabolic acidemia. After obtaining an arterial blood gas to evaluate acid-base balance, metabolic acidemia requires correction at once with sodium bicarbonate or THAM. Empirically, sodium bicarbonate (0.5-1.0 mEq/Kg IV) may be given prior to the availability of lab data, if the spell has been protracted.

The next stages of intervention involve manipulation of systemic vascular resistance or infundibular contractility in order to establish a more favorable physiological balance:

(1) Propranolol (Inderal) .05-0.1 mg/kg may be given IV cautiously, in an attempt to decrease infundibular obstruction. Long term oral therapy with propranolol has been beneficial in some patients, but is not generally recommended, today, when early surgery is available. Note, whereas propranolol may be beneficial, Digoxin is essentially contra-indicated in this group of patients.

(2) Phenylephrine (Neosynephrine) .02 mg/kg IV followed by 2-5 mcg/kg continuous IV drip, may reverse a protracted spell by increasing systemic vascular resistance. Methoxamine (Vasoxyl) 0.1 mg/kg IV may be used instead of phenylephrine to acutely increase systemic vascular resistance.

(3) Intubation with controlled ventilation (muscle paralysis) as well as possible emergency palliative surgery are rarely necessary for intractable situations.

<u>Summary</u>: Although severe hypercyanotic spells in infants and children with certain congenital heart defects are now rare because of early surgery, they must be treated immediately and efficiently. They have the rare potential of causing death. Parents should be given instructions for initial stages of therapy and shown how to perform knee-chest positioning. Therapy includes:

(1) Knee-chest positioning (intermittent)
(2) 100% oxygen administration
(3) Morphine sulfate 0.1-0.2 mg/kg IV or SC
(4) Propranolol .05-0.1 mg/kg IV with caution
(5) Phenylephrine .02 mg/kg IV followed by 2-5 mcg/kg/min continuous IV drip
(6) Methoxamine 0.1 mg/kg IV may be used in lieu of the initial dose of phenylephrine
(7) Intubation with controlled ventilation (including muscle paralysis), as well as possible emergency palliative surgery are indicated for intractable hypercyanotic spells.

CARDIAC DYSRHYTHMIAS

Along with pediatric ECG interpretation, the most difficult challenge to the house officer in Pediatrics or Family Practice, is a logical approach to interpretation and early management of the basic pediatric dysrhythmias. Importantly, it is not common for a dysrhythmia in the pediatric patient to be unstable enough as to become life threatening, although this is rarely the case. By far the most common dysrhythmias are either premature supraventricular or ventricular beats. With a little experience the physician should be able to suspect premature beats by noting their earlier than usual appearance in an otherwise regular rhythm. The ECG determines the source of premature beat as supraventricular or ventricular, ordinarily, although junctional premature beats conducted aberrantly cannot be easily distinguished from ventricular premature beats. Appreciation of a preceding P wave, even if hidden within the T wave, indicates that the premature beat is atrial in origin. It is quite common for the preceding P wave to be inverted in the inferior leads II, III, and AVF indicating a low atrial origin to the premature atrial beat. Presence of premature atrial or ventricular beats is ordinarily a benign phenomenon especially if an increased heart rate in response to exercise abolishes or significantly decreases the ectopy. Holter monitor demonstration of significant periods of supraventricular tachycardia may prompt therapy, although even these episodes may be tolerated well.

Fascinating variations of the isolated premature atrial or ventricular beats are the parasystolic rhythms where one is dealing with a very regular automatic atrial or ventricular focus that allows interruption of a regular rhythm only during safe periods of excitation. Detection of such a focus requires noticing that the premature ventricular beats are not consistently coupled to the last normal beat with a rather narrow coupling interval, but rather that one can determine a regular interval between the premature ventricular beats with variation of only 10% of the cycle length. In looking at a ventricular parasystole, one also often notices areas of fusion between the normal QRS complex and the parasystolic ventricular complex. If one is able to determine that a rhythm is parasystolic in nature it is very comforting, because such rhythms are very stable and require no therapy, even if the parasystolic rhythm becomes parasystolic ventricular tachycardia. We believe that the same is true of atrial parasystolic rhythms, but these are so rare in children that we cannot be certain.

A ventricular or junctional origin to a dysrhythmia is best suspected by noting dissociation between the premature beat and the intrinsic ventricular response other than the premature beat. That is, one is often able to identify non-conducted P waves in the presence of ventricular premature beats or ventricular tachycardia. A dysrhythmia as significant as ventricular tachycardia, defined as more than three ectopic ventricular beats in succession, may be well tolerated in the child with an otherwise normal heart. Over time however, most of these dysrhythmias become associated with a myopathic dysfunction and require therapy. Sudden death may occur in as many as 12.5% of symptomatic children with untreated ventricular tachycardia who otherwise have no major cardiac abnormality (5). Therapy in all children with ventricular tachycardia [excluding the children with parasystolic ventricular tachycardia who do not appear to require therapy] remains slightly controversial, nevertheless, with previous recent data suggesting little risk in 26 children followed 1 month to 34 years [mean 59 months, median 42 months]. That study reported no episode of sudden death although 2 patients were lost to follow-up (6). Phenytoin, propranolol, and quinidine are often useful in therapy of pediatric ventricular dysrhythmias. Early attempted control of ventricular tachycardia is often possible with intravenous lidocaine, but may require cardioversion in the unstable patient who may become hypotensive. Patients with prolonged QT intervals on their resting or provoked ECG [vagal maneuver or exercise] in association with any history of dizziness or syncope or documented ventricular tachycardia, must be placed on vigorous therapy with phenytoin and/or propranolol. Rarely such patients require sympathectomy for control of symptoms. Importantly this group is at risk of sudden death from disorganized ventricular tachycardia and fibrillation. In the patient with cardiomyopathy or resistant ventricular dysrhythmia, amiodarone now appears to be the drug of choice. Amiodarone given to a patient with cardiomyopathy even without a ventricular dysrhythmia, also appears very helpful in symptomatic relief.

Another very important group of patients with ventricular dysrhythmias are post operative tetralogy of Fallot patients. Garson et al (7) suggest control of any ventricular ectopy appearing in these patients as a means of decreasing risk of sudden death. Control was usually possible using phenytoin. Other centers treat only patients with greater than 30 premature ventricular beats/hour on two holter monitoring sessions, provided no couplets or triplets are present. Control of ventricular dysrhythmias was possible with dilantin, quinidine with procainamide, or amiodarone.

Supraventricular tachycardia is usually well tolerated in the older child but becomes associated with CHF in the younger infant less than 6-12 months old, if sustained longer than 24-48 hours. In these instances the child is often brought to the pediatrician for evaluation of decreased activity, easy tiring with feeding, pallor, and irritability, the classical symptoms of CHF in the infant.

Detection of heart rates greater than 200 beats/minute essentially allows the diagnosis of significant dysrhythmia, which is usually supraventricular in origin. Rarely, in children with Wolff-Parkinson-White pre-excitation syndrome, the tachycardia may show wide QRS complexes. However, usually during tachycardia these children conduct anterograde through the normal A-V nodal pathways and retrograde through the bundle of Kent, which results in a narrow QRS complex. If a question exists as to whether the tachycardia is ventricular or supraventricular in origin, immediate cardiac consultation is necessary and therapy is safest assuming a ventricular origin first. Immediate therapy of supraventricular tachycardia in infants and children less than one year of age involves rapid intravenous digitalization. If serious cardiac compromise is present with overt CHF, cardioversion with .25 - 2.0 joules [watt-sec]/Kg, is necessary. Although generally safe to further maintain the infant and child with Wolff-Parkinson-White [WPW] syndrome on chronic digoxin therapy, it is important to realize that such patients often require additional or alternative therapy with agents such as propranolol. In the adult population, digoxin is essentially contra-indicated in patients with WPW because it may promote one to one conduction along the Kent bundle in face of atrial flutter, and may under these circumstances result in ventricular fibrillation. Studies in children support the safe use of Digoxin in face of WPW in most instances although some children behave electrophysiologically like the adult group with WPW. Fortunately atrial flutter is rare in children. In the older child with supraventricular tachycardia who is not compromised functionally, intravenous verapamil now appears to be the therapy of choice [0.15 mg/Kg over one minute and repeated once in 20 minutes if necessary]. Beware of A-V block after administration of verapamil ranging from first to second degree block, usually. In well controlled European studies intravenous Adenosine Triphosphate [ATP] appeared superior to verapamil and digoxin in the immediate conversion of PST (8). It is very vagomimetic and has a very short half-life. A very recent study in this country suggests that adenosine itself may be even better for conversion of PST and has less side effects compared with ATP. Administration of rapid intravenous 37.5 mcg/Kg doses of adenosine every two minutes until termination of tachycardia or development of A-V block, demonstrated that the usual minimum effective total dose range was 131 +/- 77 mcg/Kg, with minimal side effects such as transient dyspnea (9). A very short acting intravenous beta blocking agent may also prove useful in these patients, and should be released in this country very soon [Breviblock (esmolol by Dupont Critical Care)].

The above dysrhythmias are usually considered re-entrant in nature; however, another entire group of pediatric dysrhythmias is now considered automatic in nature [apart from the concepts of parasystole]. These dysrhythmias may prove to be the most difficult to manage, especially the atrial ectopic tachycardias which are difficult to suspect in the otherwise normal child. However, appreciation of a third heart sound or summation gallop is often possible in such instances. The author has had two patients with ectopic supraventricular tachycardias: one with a junctional focus responded well to oral verapamil, whereas the one with an atrial ectopic focus responded very well to maintenance amiodarone after showing response to intravenous amiodarone during electrophysiological studies. It appears from early experience that some of the resistant ectopic or automatic atrial tachycardias may be responsive to amiodarone therapy (10), although others may require electrical or surgical ablation. Amiodarone has many significant side effects in adults, but thus far has not been associated with similar side effects in the child. Pulmonary fibrosis, thyroid abnormalities, corneal densities, and grey skin discoloration are possible in the adult, but only corneal opacities have been noted in children, and these are reversible upon discontinuation of the drug. Early results with ethmozine, another new antidysrhythmic drug, are also favorable in the treatment of automatic atrial tachycardia. This drug has the advantage of much less side effects compared with amiodarone, although as noted above, amiodarone in children appears quite safe, thus far.

Another important group of dysrhythmias is the group involving interruption of usual conduction of impulse formation. Congenital complete heart block is a perfect example of this group. Beware that there is a high association of maternal systemic Lupus Erythematosis in association with congenital complete heart block. Although tolerated quite well in most instances, children born with complete heart block associated with rates less than 45-50 beat/min usually require permanent pacemaker implantation. Persistent surgically induced complete heart block is now more rare, but requires permanent pacemaker therapy also. Second degree A-V block is not very common in children and ordinarily is benign without progression to complete A-V block. Amongst the only exceptions to this are children with otherwise uncomplicated corrected transposition [L-loop/ isolated ventricular inversion] who are at risk of late development of complete heart block and require careful monitoring. First degree A-V block is common in children with isolated ASD, VSD, with endocardial cushion defects and associated with digoxin therapy. It is not a sign of toxicity but rather of effect in regard to digoxin therapy. When prevalent, children with acute rheumatic fever often developed first degree A-V block. PR interval prolongation may also be familial and is benign under those circumstances. In association with surgically induced bifascicular block [right and left anterior bundles], the presence of first degree A-V block requires further careful evaluation, including electrophysiological studies, because of the possible development of serious complete heart block with possible sudden death.

Sick sinus syndrome associated with both brady and tachydysrhythmias, is fortunately rare in children but may occur. Very slow sinus rates found in the trained athlete are most often normal, although somewhat disturbing to the examining physician.

Common sense must prevail in work up of pediatric dysrhythmias. Those with a history of daily or very frequent occurrence may be documented on a standard ECG or 24 hour holter monitoring, usually. Those provoked by activity are usually elaborated upon ECG stress testing, and those that are rare may be documented by the newer transtelephonic ECG recorders. Only after documentation of the dysrhythmia is logical therapy possible. History is also important. If the patient notes that there is a sudden start and halt to the rapid, pounding dysrhythmia, it is most often PST. A feeling of dizziness or nausea is common in prolonged episodes of PST. Cardiac dysrhythmias are often familial and often associated with mitral and/or tricuspid valve prolapse. Echocardiographic evaluation is essential in all forms of dysrhythmias in order to rule out cardiomyopathy and tumors. Neonatal myofibromata may present with atrial dysrhythmias. Dysrhythmias associated with previous cardiac surgery, cardiomyopathy, or myocarditis are the most serious and require very careful evaluation and therapy at a center able to perform sophisticated pediatric electrophysiological studies, overdrive suppression with temporary pacemakers, and implantation of permanent pacemakers if necessary. Balloon counterpulsation support could become necessary in the extremely ill child with ventricular dysrhythmia secondary to myocarditis.

Table 7.2 lists doses of pediatric drugs used for cardiac dysrhythmias, including newer experimental drugs (11). It is important to realize that these drugs should not be used without the supervision of a qualified pediatric cardiologist, preferably with experience in complex pediatric dysrhythmias. For drugs not listed, one could estimate pediatric doses using body surface area [BSA] ratios. As presented in Chapter 3:

BSA [m²] = 0.024265 x H^.3964 x W^.5378, where H=Height(cm), W=Weight(kg), and ^="raised to the power of" (12).

If one assumes normal adult BSA as 1.7, estimated pediatric dosage would be [Child's BSA/1.7] x adult standard dose (13).

Table 7.2: Drug Dosages and Indications in Therapy of Pediatric Cardiac Dysrhythmias

Acebutolol [Sectral]:

DOSE: 10 - 25 mg/kg/day in 2 divided doses with maximum dose of 200-400 mg bid

USE: The author has had much experience with this cardioselective beta blocking agent which has been particularly important in a patient with hypertrophic obstructive cardiomyopathy and asthma as well as WPW syndrome. No significant wheezing has occurred for at least five years of chronic therapy. This drug has also been useful in control of PST in a child with WPW syndrome and asthma as well. Should not be used in patients with cardiac failure, and care must still be taken in patients with asthma.

Amiodarone [Cordarone]:

DOSE: 5 mg/Kg/dose p.o. twice daily for 10 days; then 5-7 mg/Kg/day. Try to taper slowly over periods of 4-6 months to 2.5-4.0 mg/Kg/day if dysrhythmia does not recur.

IV dose is 3-6 mg/Kg but this must be given only under completely controlled conditions either in the cath lab or intensive care unit.

USES: Refractory ventricular dysrhythmias including ventricular tachycardia, especially in children with cardiomyopathy. Refractory atrial dysrhythmias including atrial flutter, supraventricular tachycardia, and automatic or ectopic atrial tachycardia.

Aprinidine (Group Ia):

DOSE: PO 1.5 mg/kg every 6 hours first day; 1.0 mg/kg every six hour second day; 0.75 mg/kg every six hours third day; then 0.3-0.75 mg/kg/dose every 8-12 hours.

USE: Serious refractory atrial or ventricular dysrhythmias.

Atropine Sulfate:

DOSE: IV or subcutaneous .01-.03 mg/kg/dose with maximum dose 0.4 mg every 4-6 hours.

USES: Vagally mediated bradycardias, including digitalis related bradycardia. May produce hypotension and flushing.

Bretylium tosylate [Bretylol] (Group IV):

DOSE: IV 5 mg/kg/bolus q 6 h up to 48 hours.

USES: Stabilization of ventricular tachycardia/ fibrillation after unsuccessful cardioversion. Aggravates digitalis toxicity.

Digitalis [Lanoxin]:

DOSE: See Chapter 7, p 143.

USES: Conversion and maintenance therapy for paroxysmal supraventricular tachycardia. Beware of use in older children and adults with WPW.

Diphenylhydantoin [Dilantin] (Group Ib):

DOSE: IV 3-5 mg/Kg over 5 minutes. Oral Dose is 2-5 mg/Kg/day divided into 2-3 doses. Small changes in oral doses may have marked effects on serum level in the patient receiving chronic medication and in steady state.

USES: Simple ventricular dysrhythmias. May be combined with disopyramide [Norpace]. May be used alone in patients with prolonged QT interval syndrome and ventricular tachycardia. [Norpace is contraindicated in such patients.]

Disopyramide [Norpace] (Group Ia):

DOSE: IV 1.5-2.5 mg/Kg slowly. Orally 2-6 mg/Kg/day in four divided doses. Has considerable anticholinergic effect.

USES: Ventricular dysrhythmias. Depresses myocardial function and *should not* be used in patients with prolonged QT interval syndrome as with other class I agents.

Encainide :

DOSE: 60-120 mg/m^2/day divided into 6-8 hour doses. Some centers list dosage as 1-3 mg/kg/day in four divided dose p.o.

USES: Permanent junctional reciprocating tachycardia. Other supraventricular dysrhythmias refractory to digoxin, propranolol, or verapamil, including reciprocating AV tachycardia, chaotic atrial tachycardia [one infant also had WPW syndrome]. Proarrhythmic effect [new or worsening dysrhythmias] are possible with this drug. May be combined with verapamil or propranolol.

Ethmozine:

DOSE: 200 $mg/m^2/day$ to maximum of 600 $mg/m^2/day$ divided into three doses/day.

USES: Automatic atrial tachycardia, junctional ectopic tachycardia, permanent junctional reciprocating tachycardia.

Isoproterenol [Isuprel]:

DOSES: IV .05-.4 micrograms/Kg/min as a 4 mg/liter drip.

USES: Cardiopulmonary resuscitation where bradycardia is present. Bradycardia that is not vagally mediated.

Lidocaine [xylocaine] {Group Ib}:

DOSE: IV 0.5-1.0 mg/Kg/dose every 20-60 min PRN.

USES: Initial stabilization of serious ventricular tachycardia.

Mexiletine [Mexitil} {Group Ib}:

DOSE: 1.4-5.1 mg/Kd/dose every eight hours.

USES: Ventricular tachycardia, ventricular couplets, multiform ventricular premature beats, and uniform premature ventricular beats, including patients with cardiomyopathy and arrhythmogenic right ventricular dysplasia. Response appears poor in patients with cardiomyopathy and normal hearts, but good in post-operative dysrhythmias.

Nadolol [Corgard] {Group III}:

DOSE: 0.5 - 2.5 mg/kg/dose once daily. Available in 40 mg and 80 mg scored tablets but 20 mg tablets are also available for investigational purposes.

USES: Preliminary data suggests that a once daily dose of Nadolol is useful for atrial and ventricular dysrhythmias already shown to be controlled by propranolol in a given patient. These dysrhythmias include PST and ventricular tachycardia (14).

Procainamide [Pronestyl] {Group Ia}:

DOSE: IV 10-100 mg/kg as slow diluted drip over 5 minutes, repeated PRN every 10-30 minutes. PO 40-60 mg/kg/day in 4-6 divided doses.

USES: Ventricular dysrhythmias, usually responding to lidocaine IV, initially.

Propafenone:

DOSE: 0.2 mg/Kg/iv bolus repeated every 10 minutes to a maximum of 2 mg/Kg/iv bolus. Once ventricular rate decreases below 150 BPM, continuous infusion is started at 4-7 micrograms/kg/min. Colloid infusion may be necessary for hypotensive effects. AV sequential pacing is usually necessary to restore AV synchrony.

USES: Life threatening post-operative junctional ectopic tachycardia [JET].

Propranolol [Inderal] {Group II}:

DOSE: IV .01-.15 mg/kg/dose slowly over 10 minutes with careful blood pressure and ECG monitoring for bradycardia or hypotension; may repeat q6-8 hours PRN with care. PO 0.5 - 1.0 mg/kg/dose given every 6 hours [total daily dose of 4 mg/kg/day].

USES: Paroxysmal supraventricular tachycardia, especially associated with WPW syndrome, ventricular dysrhythmias. Uses in cardiac problems other than dysrhythmias include panic attack syndrome, pain associated with mitral valve prolapse, relief of subaortic obstruction in patients with hypertrophic obstructive cardiomyopathy. Contraindicated in patients with reactive airway disease such as asthma. Newer cardioselective agents may be useful in this group.

Quinidine gluconate {Group Ia}:

DOSE: PO 10-30 mg/kg/day [e.g., 160-660 mg every 12 hours]

USES: Ventricular dysrhythmias. Atrial dysrhythmias that may be associated with WPW syndrome, although quinidine is rarely necessary with newer drugs available.

Quinidine sulfate {Group Ia}:

DOSE: PO 3-6 mg/kg/dose every 2-3 hours 5 times daily for a maximum dose of 12 mg/kg/dose every 2-3 hours 5 times daily.

USES: As for quinidine gluconate.

Tocainide [Tonocard] {Group Ib}:

DOSE: PO 6-8 mg/kg/dose given every 8-12 hours

USE: Serious ventricular dysrhythmias.

Verapamil [Isoptin, Calan] {Group IV}:

DOSE: IV 0.1-0.2 mg/kg over 1 minute, repeated once in 30 minutes. PO 3-6 mg/kg/day divided into 3 doses. May be suspended in an acid medium such as USP Cherry Syrup with a one month shelf life.

USES: Termination of PST, rapidly in children over 1 year of age. As with digitalis, *do not use in older patients with WPW or other pre-excitation conduction*. May be useful in ectopic junctional tachycardia and other forms of PST.

PERICARDIAL DISEASE

Clinical suspicion of pericarditis with large pericardial effusion or early tamponade is critical in order to intervene prior to serious cardiac tamponade. Patients presenting with acute pericarditis most often complain of significant precordial chest pain which may be referred to the epigastrium, shoulder, neck or left arm. They are often restless if a large pericardial effusion or early tamponade is present, preferring to be in a sitting position rather than a recumbent position. Deep inspiration usually worsens the pain. With large effusions, precordial cardiac activity is decreased, although one is usually able to determine the position of the apical impulse. If the patient is older, one will be able to percuss the left border of cardiac dullness quite lateral with respect to the apical impulse. This finding suggested a clinical diagnosis of pericardial effusion in days prior to echocardiography. Heart sounds are distant or diminished, and one is able to appreciate a pericardial friction rub if the effusion is not too large. ECG changes with acute pericarditis include early ST segment elevation followed after 1-2 weeks, by T-wave flattening and/or inversion. Echocardiographic diagnosis is almost always definitive, whereas radiographs of the chest may only demonstrate non-specific cardiac enlargement.

The most feared consequence of pericardial disease is effusion or constriction progressing to cardiac tamponade. Signs of tamponade include increasing restlessness, marked discomfort upon reclining, hyperpnea or dyspnea, increased jugular venous pulsations, tachycardia, hepatomegaly with a sharp liver margin [if the event is very acute and not associated with congestive cardiac failure], peripheral vasoconstriction with decreased peripheral pulses. *Pulsus paradoxus* may develop whereby one is able to appreciate a greater than 10 mm Hg decrease in systolic pressure during quiet inspiration. Paradoxically increased jugular venous pressure during inspiration [Kussmaul sign] may also develop with severe tamponade. These physical signs of tamponade are very important, because echocardiographic findings of tamponade may be somewhat non-specific, although as noted it is extremely important in the detection of pericardial effusion. Unless there is a known definitive etiology for the effusion such as postpericardiotomy syndrome, one must perform pericardiocentesis for culture to include tuberculous and fungal origins. There are many methods for pericardiocentesis; However, the most common is to aseptically insert a long #20 spinal or pericardial needle just to the left of the xiphoid process, pointing to the left shoulder at an angle of 30° toward the patient's back. The patient should be in a sitting or 45° upright position so that pericardial fluid is dependent. Insert the needle only as far as necessary to drain pericardial fluid or obtain samples for culture and possible cell block preparation. One usually attaches a precordial ECG lead to this exploring needle in order to detect any myocardial current of injury, indicating that the needle is touching the myocardium and that no further entry should occur. Another useful approach is to guide needle insertion by echocardiography. This procedure should not be done unless the patient is in an intensive care unit or well equipped cardiac cath lab. Furthermore, surgical intervention should be immediately available should surgical drainage of the effusion be necessary or should a significant complication to pericardiocentesis occur, such as injury to a vascular structure or the heart, resulting in rapid bleeding.

Pyogenic pericarditis may occur in association with staphyloccocci [usually *S. aureus*], *Streptococcus pneumoniae*, *Haemophilus influenzae*, *Neisseria meningitidis*, and other streptococci. Other causes importantly include *M. tuberculosis*, *E. coli*, pseudomonas, gonococci, *Klebsiella*, *Proteus*, and bacteroides. *M. tuberculosis* may cause very significant late constrictive pericarditis, requiring pericardiectomy, when possible. Fever and leukocytosis is common with pyogenic pericarditis, whereas the patient with viral pericarditis appears less toxic, generally has a lower grade fever, and a normal white count or elevation in lymphocyte count. Pulmonary infiltrates and pleural effusions may also occur in viral pericarditis.

Other miscellaneous causes of pericarditis with or without effusion, include lupus erythematosis, juvenile rheumatoid arthritis where pericardial effusions are often massive, malignant tumors, uremia, chronic anemias such as sickle cell disease, thalassemia and congenital aplastic anemia, myxedema, gout, chest irradiation, drugs such as practolol, hydralazine, and procainamide, blunt or penetrating thoracic trauma associated with hemopericardium, acute rheumatic fever, and postpericardiotomy syndrome. Rarely an effusion is chylous if injury to the thoracic duct occurred during surgical manipulation.

Postpericardiotomy syndrome occurs in approximately 25-30% of children undergoing open heart surgery or palliative procedures requiring incision of the pericardium. It can begin as early as three days after a procedure or as late as 3-4 weeks after a procedure. Fever, chest pain, and cough are usual. Congestive cardiac failure may accompany this syndrome and signs of pericardial tamponade may occur if the effusion is expanding quickly. All patients have high heart reactive antibody titers and 70% demonstrate an acute increase in antibodies to such viruses as adenovirus, Coxsackie B, or cytomegalovirus.

Treatment of purulent pericariditis involves systemic antibiotic therapy as well as possible surgical relief of the effusion if constriction or tamponade develop. Loculation of the effusion may occur, making antibiotic therapy less helpful, and surgical drainage usually necessary. Indwelling pericardial catheters may also be necessary for cases resistant to usual therapy.

Aspirin [120 mg/Kg/day divided into 4 or 6 daily doses] is extremely useful in the therapy of postpericardiotomy syndrome, and is also helpful in non-specific or viral pericarditis. Continuation of aspirin therapy is often necessary for as long as 6 weeks with postpericardiotomy syndrome, because earlier tapering or discontinuation may result in recurrence. Tapering of aspirin doses at the end of therapy with or without the addition of steroid therapy may avoid rebound as well. Bed rest is very important. Occasionally steroids are necessary in patients with severe postpericardiotomy syndrome but likely should not be used in patients with acute viral pericarditis, unless symptoms become recurrent or protracted and severe. Indomethacin is often useful in cases of non-specific recurrent pericarditis or with postpericardiotomy syndrome as well.

CARDIOPULMONARY RESUSCITATION

Recommendations for pediatric cardiopulmonary resuscitation [CPR] often change according to current American Heart Association CPR course material, for which reason the topic will not be covered in detail. The basic admonition of attention to airway, breathing, and circulation applies to infants and children as well as the adult. Mouth to mouth, or bag and mask ventilation are possible once the airway is cleared, but intubation is preferable, with subsequent use of bag ventilation. Recommended ventilatory rates are 20/min in the infant and 15/min in the child. One may estimate necessary endotracheal tube size [French] using the formula: SIZE = [Age (years) + 16]/4

Generally, the tube is similar in diameter to the child's fifth finger.

Cardiac massage frequency should be 100/min in the infant and 80/min in the child with a compression to breath ratio of 5:1. Three fingers are usually adequate to compress the infant, whereas the heel of the hand may be used in the older child. Depth of compression should be .5 to 1 inch in the infant and 1 to 1.5 inches in the older child.

Immediate venous access is important but intratracheal administration of many drugs is possible including epinephrine. Recent data suggest that compression duration is more important than rate and should represent at least 50% of the cycle time. Interestingly this implies that higher rates of compression [80-90/min] used in children may also be useful in the adult to provide a relatively longer duration. Flow to the brain is thought to result from transmitted intrathoracic pressure during compression aided by maintaining carotid vascular tone by drugs such as epinephrine. Interesting observations in the cath lab indicate that patients suffering from ventricular fibrillation or asystole can maintain adequate cerebral blood flow to prevent loss of consciousness by coughing at least 40-60 times/min. Theoretically the cough increased intrathoracic pressure adequately to transmit adequate cerebral blood flow (15).

In infants and children, correction of metabolic acidosis with sodium bicarbonate is important. *Those patients receiving digoxin should not receive intravenous boluses of calcium gluconate or chloride* because of the risk of ventricular asystole.

Drugs useful in resuscitation include:

Amrinone [Inocor] 0.5 to 1.0 mg/kg IV q 15-30 minutes as inotropic agent other than catecholamine group.

Atropine .01 to .02 mg/kg dose IV with maximum dose of 0.4 mg. May repeat low dose twice in 60 minutes.

Bretylium tosylate 5 mg/kg as IV bolus prior to attempted defibrillation or cardioversion in intractable ventricular dysrhythmias.

Calcium gluconate [10% solution] 0.6 ml/kg to 10 ml/dose IV [*beware of use in digitalized patients*]

Dobutamine [Dobutrex] 2-10 mcg/kg/min by continuous IV infusion.

Dopamine 2-5 mcg/kg/min increased slowly according to need by 5-10 mcg/Kg/min increments after a 15 minute trial on each dose by continuous IV infusion with maximum of 25 mcg/Kg/min.

Epinephrine [1:10,000 dilution] 0.1 ml/kg IV in the infant and empirically 1-5 ml] IV in the older child. May give by intracardiac or intratracheal routes.

Epinephrine [1:1000 dilution for continuous infusion] 0.1 to 1.0 mcg/kg/min by continuous IV infusion.

Isoproterenol 0.1 to 1.0 mcg/kg/min by continuous IV infusion.

Levarterenol 0.1 mcg/kg/min by continuous IV infusion, not to exceed 1.0 mcg/Kg/min.

Naloxone [Narcan] 5-10 mcg/kg/dose repeated every 2-3 minutes as needed with maximum of 400 mcg/dose in the older child.

Sodium Bicarbonate 1-3 mEq/kg IV as necessary to correct metabolic acidosis.

Defibrillation energy is 2.2 joules/kg or 1 joule/pound.

Cardioversion energy is .5 to 2.2 joules/kg or .25 to 1 joule/pound.

GENERAL READING

Dillon TR, Janos GG, Meyer RA, Benzing III GB, Kaplan S: Vasodilator therapy for congestive heart failure. *J Peds* 96:623, 1980.

Gillette PC, Garson A (eds): *Pediatric Cardiac Dysrhythmias*. New York, Grune & Stratton Publishing Co, Inc., 1981.

Linday LA, Engle MA: Prostaglandin treatment of newborns with ductal-dependent congenital heart disease. *Pediatr Ann* 10(4):29-38, 1981.

Moss AJ, Adams FH, Emmanouillides GC: *Heart Disease in Infants, Children and Adolescents*, Third Edition. Baltimore, The Williams & Wilkins Co, 1983.

Orlowski JP: Cardiopulmonary Resuscitation in Children. *Ped Clin N Amer* 27(3):495-513, 1980.

Roberts NK, Gelband H (eds): *Cardiac Arrhythmias in the Neonate, Infant, and Child*. New York, Appleton-Century-Crofts, 1977.

Rudolph, AM: *Congenital Diseases of the Heart*. Chicago, Year Book, 1974.

Rudolph AM (ed): *Pediatrics*, Seventeenth Edition. Norwalk, Appleton-Century-Crofts, 1982.

Veasy LG, Orsmond GS, Ruttenbeg HD, Boucek MM: Pediatric use of intraaortic balloon pumping (abstract). Presented at the Twenty-Fifth Annual Meeting of the Cardiology Section (American Academy of Pediatrics), San Francisco, October, 1983.

Notes

1. Sacks EJ et al: Diagnosis and Therapy of Pediatric Cardiac Emergencies (Chapter 22). In Chung EK [ed]: *Cardiac Emergencies*, Third Edition. Philadelphia, Lee & Febiger, 1985 [With Permission].

2. Park MK: Use of digoxin in infants and children, with specific emphasis on dosage. *J Pediatrics* 108: 871-877, 1986.

3. Sacks EJ et al: Diagnosis and Therapy of Pediatric Cardiac Emergencies (Chapter 22). In Chung EK [ed]: *Cardiac Emergencies*, Third Edition. Philadelphia, Lee & Febiger, 1985 [With Permission].

4. Ibid.

5. Deal BJ, Miller SM, Scagliotti D, Prechel D, Gallastegui JL, Hariman RJ: Ventricular tachycardia in a young population without overt heart disease. *Circulation* 73:1111-1118, 1986.

6. Fulton DR, Chung KJ, Tabakin BS, Keane JF: Ventricular Tachycardia in Children Without Heart Disease. *Am J Cardiol* 55:1328-1331, 1985.

7. Garson A Jr, Randall DC, Gillette PC, Smith RT, Moak JP, McVey P, McNamara DG: Prevention of Sudden Death After Repair of Tetralogy of Fallot: Treatment of Ventricular Arrhythmias. *JACC* 6:221-227, 1985.

8. Greco R, et al: Treatment of paroxysmal supraventricular tachycardia in infancy with Digitalis, Adenosine-5′-Triphosphate, and Verapamil: A Comparative Study. *Circulation* 66:504-508, 1982.

9. Overholt ED, et al: The use of adenosine in children with supraventricular tachycardia. AAP abstract. *Am Heart J* 112:648, 1986.

10. Mehta AV, Ewing L, Sacks EJ, Balian A, Sanchez G: "Automatic Ectopic Atrial Tachycardia in Children: Is Ablation Needed?". Presented at American College of Cardiology Annual Meetings, Atlanta. March 11, 1986

11. Moak JP: Newer Antiarrhythmic Drugs in Pediatrics. *Cardio* p 45-49, June,1986.

12. Haycock GB, Schwartz GJ, Wisotsky DH: Geometric method for measuring body surface area: A height-weight formula validated in infants, children, and adults. *J Peds* 93:62, 1978

13. Garson A: Dosing the Newer Antiarrhythmic Drugs in Children: Consideration in Pediatric Pharmacology [Editorial]. *Am J Cardiol* 57:1405–1407, 1986.

14. Mehta AV: Personal communication, October, 1986.

15. Weisfeldt ML, Halperin HR: Cardiopulmonary resuscitation: beyond massage. *Circulation* 74:443–448, 1986.

Chapter 8

Kawasaki Disease and Acute Rheumatic Fever

KAWASAKI DISEASE [Mucocutaneous Lymph Node Syndrome]

As acute rheumatic fever has declined significantly, Kawasaki Disease [KD] has increased significantly in this country, after its first description from Japan in 1967. Etiology remains unknown. Most cases occur in late winter and early spring in the United States and Canada. Prevalence in non-epidemic years is estimated as 1.6-5.6/100,000 children increasing to 13.5-16.4/100,000 during epidemics. Average estimates of annual incidence in the United States is 3,000-3,500 children/year with 600-700 developing coronary arterial abnormalities. Peak age incidence is 13-24 months with 80% of children with KD less than 4-5 years old. KD is rare in children older than 10 years and only 3-4 cases older than 14 years have been reported to the Center for Disease Control in Atlanta [CDC]. Mortality in the United States is a relatively low 0.5 to 1% [15 deaths have been reported to the Atlanta CDC between 1976-84], and mostly secondary to thrombosis of coronary arterial aneurysms, which occur in about 20% of children with KD. Fortunately these dominantly proximal coronary arterial aneurysms are amendable to cross sectional echocardiographic evaluation and most resolve uneventfully. Children of Asian descent less than 4-5 years old are 6 times more susceptible and Black children are 1.5 times more susceptible compared with caucasian children. There is also a 1.4:1.0 male to female ratio.

Similar to the process used in making a diagnosis of acute rheumatic fever, one must rely upon a set of criteria in order to make a sensible diagnosis of KD in children. The six findings associated with KD include:

[1] prolonged fever lasting 5 or more days;

[2] conjunctival congestion;

[3] oral cavity mucous membrane changes including erythema, dryness, angular fissuring of the lips, erythema

of the tongue with prominence of the papillae, diffuse reddening of the oropharyngeal mucosa:

[4] erythema and induration of the hands and feet with membranous periungal desquamation:

[5] non-specific or polymorphous exanthem;

[6] cervical nonsuppurative lymphadenitis.

Five out of the six above criteria or four of the above criteria in face of prolonged fever, allow the diagnosis of KD. Shortly after the onset of high fever, during the first week of the illness, conjunctival involvement, cracked red lips, erythematous buccal mucosa, strawberry tongue, and cervical adenitis may appear. Between 15-25 days, marked thrombocytosis occurs. By the beginning and middle of the second week of illness erythema followed by edema of the hands and feet, and a polymorphous exanthem develop. By the middle of the third week of illness peeling of the tips of the fingers and toes followed by the palms and soles, occurs. Creasing of nails may occur by the middle of the second month from the start of the illness. Irritability is marked and very common.

CDC [Atlanta] reports the following incidence of cardiac complications: Coronary aneurysms [19%: note that there is a 0.2% incidence of aneurysms in other blood vessels], myocarditis [10.1%], pericardial effusion [5.1%], myocardial ischemia [3.6%], dysrhythmias [3.4%], CHF [1.5%], myocardial infarction 0.9%], abnormal ECG [16%]. Aortic and/or mitral insufficiency also occur acutely.

Other systemic involvement includes: Arthritis/arthralgia [27%], meatitis/sterile pyuria [9.8%], hepatitis [8%], aseptic meningitis [7%], myalgia/myositis [3.6%], hydrops of the gallbladder [2.9%], iritis/uveitis [1.3%] (1).

Therapy consists of therapeutic levels of aspirin during the acute stages of KD [see study below, using gammaglobulin]. Interestingly, doses higher than the 100-110 mg/Kg/day range may be necessary in children with KD, in order to achieve serum salicylate levels in the 20 mg% range (2). Thrombocytosis and erythrocyte sedimentation rates may be monitored as a guide to discontinuation of salicylate therapy. However, children in whom coronary arterial aneurysms develop require long term low dose [3-5 mg/Kg/day] until echocardiographic evidence of aneurysm resolution occurs. Dipyridamole [persantine] 25-50 mg 1-3 times/day [about 5 mg/Kg/day] may be used to augment the salicylate antiplatelet effect, but studies of its use are not complete, and appropriate dosing is not completely known. The issue of using salicylates in face of public concern over Reye syndrome has been eloquently addressed by Drs. Takahashi and Mason (3), who indicate that the chance of concomitant development of KD and Reye syndrome is extremely low. Good practice would nevertheless suggest that a child on chronic salicylate therapy may be best maintained with dipyridamole in lieu of salicylates during episodes of influenza or varicella. Use of large dose intravenous gammaglobulin therapy in addition to aspirin therapy to prevent coronary arterial aneurysms remains investigational (4). However, there is now a recently completed multicenter controlled study involving 84 children with KD who received high dose gamma globulin [400 mg/kg/day over 2 hours on 4 consecutive days, *started within 10 days of initial fever*] compared with 84 children with KD who did not receive gamma globulin [GG]. Both groups received appropriate aspirin therapy as well [80-120 mg/kg/day aspirin given in divided doses every six hours for the first 14 days of illness followed by 3-5 mg/kg/day given as one daily dose for the remainder of approximately seven weeks, unless the child had coronary arterial involvement in which case low dose aspirin continued]. Results demonstrated that the group receiving gamma globulin developed one-third less coronary abnormalities at 2 weeks after therapy [8 versus 23%] and one-fifth less coronary abnormalities at the seventh week of the study [4 versus 18%]. It is important to begin GG therapy very early in the acute course [within 10 or less days of initial fever] if used at all. The intravenous GG used in the study was manufactured by Immuno AG [Vienna, Austria], and unfortunately is not yet approved by the FDA. The study group conjecture that commercially available intravenous gamma globulins should be effective as well but the author believes that this is not completely known, and that further controlled studies are essential in the elaboration of pathogenesis and most effective therapy (5). Centers in the study do have the experimental GG available and include: Children's Hospital, Boston; Tufts-New England Medical Center, Boston; Children's Memorial Hospital, Chicago; Children's Hospital, Denver; Children's Hospital of Los Angeles; Children's Hospital and Health Center, San Diego; Kapiolani Women's and Children's Medical Center, Honolulu (6). The above study data are also interesting compared with Japanese data indicating a 6% coronary artery aneurysm incidence in children receiving only ASA therapy compared with a 5% incidence in children receiving both ASA and GG therapy by one year after initial KD (7).

An important consideration is identification of the child with increased risk of coronary arterial involvement because this group is at highest risk of serious complications and possible mortality. Results of an earlier study indicate that increased serum levels of beta-thromboglobulin [generally >43 ng/ml] may predict the group at highest risk (8). Recently Dr. Koren et al discovered that fever lasting 14 days or greater with KD was as predictive of a greater risk for coronary artery involvement as Dr. Asai's risk table (9). This study also indicated no increased risk of coronary arterial involvement in children less than 1 year old. For completeness, below is the modified Asai scoring system (10):

FINDING	SCORE 2	1	0
Age < 1 year	–	+	–
Gender	–	Male	–
Fever [days]	>/=16	14–15	</=13
ESR [mm/hr]	>/=100	60–100	<60
Elevated ESR [days]	>30	–	–
Hemoglobin <10 G%	–	+	–
Leukocyte Count [x10^9/L]	>30	26–30	<26
Arrhythmia	+	–	–
Cardiomegaly [50% C/T ratio]	–	+	–
Abnormal ECG	+	–	–

Scores equal to or greater than 6, suggest increased risk of coronary artery involvement.

The presence of new Q waves in leads I and AVL or in leads II, III, and AVF on an ECG in a patient with KD indicates myocardial fibrosis and necrosis. ECG changes also give evidence of the myocarditis associated with KD in addition to the coronary arterial involvement (11). More recent reports also indicate development of aortic and mitral insufficiency associated with KD, with both possibly becoming late sequelae (12). In Japan there is a 5% incidence of aortic and 10% incidence of mitral valve involvement, acutely (13).

Most recent data suggest that careful cardiology follow-up of these children is necessary even after the acute phase when ECHO evaluation of the proximal coronary arteries is necessary. Although risk of sudden death decreases significantly six months after the acute illness, late development of coronary aneurysms has been reported. Because aneurysm formation should be an acute pathological process, these late findings of coronary arterial aneurysms, may reflect failure of previous detection or recurrence which is possible in 0.6% of cases. The author suggests ECHO evaluation within 2 to 6 weeks of the onset of KD followed by one between 4-6 months and between 9-12 months after the illness. If no coronary aneurysms are present, further study could be delayed for several years, but should be repeated to rule out the small possibility of late development of coronary arterial aneurysms. *If coronary arterial aneurysms are present, follow up needs to be individualized.* Rarely, coronary arterial involvement is severe enough to require coronary arteriography, especially if one suspects more distal involvement. ECG at the time of ECHO would be desirable in face of evidence correlating ECG findings with coronary arterial and myocardial involvement. Much more work remains to be done relating to diagnosis, pathogenesis, and management of KD. Fascinating preliminary CDC data suggests a possible retrovirus association and also indicate that outbreaks have a proximal large body of water in common (14).

ACUTE RHEUMATIC FEVER [ARF]

Introduction: Although fortunately now uncommon, ARF remains one of the most challenging and interesting illnesses. Accurate clinical diagnosis and effective therapy still elude many younger physicians whose recent training would not include significant exposure to ARF. Diagnosis involves a broad consideration of many factors in a given patient and reflects sound knowledge of the modified Jones criteria. Etiology links specifically to antecedent Group A beta hemolytic streptoccal [GABS] pharyngitis in children predominantly between 5 and 15 years of age. ARF is very uncommon between 2 and 5 years of age and almost non-existent in children younger than 2 years of age. Most accepted theories of pathogenesis involve notions of cross reactivity between antibodies directed toward GABS and target organs such as the heart, producing pancarditis (15). In a brilliant T. Duckett Jones Memorial Lecture (16), Dr. Lewis Wannamaker jolts our complacent recent theories with the fact that there may be a component of direct cardiotoxic effects of GABS on the heart in addition to or in conjunction with the accepted autoimmune theories. He also quotes basic research findings that might explain why other areas of GABS infection such as skin [streptococcal impetigo] are not associated with ARF. There is in vitro evidence of direct cardiotoxic effects of Streptolysin-O in mammalian heart tissue cultures. What is fascinating is the fact that these effects are negated by addition of cholesterol to the tissue culture. The skin lipids of children are heavily laden with cholesterol, compared with the adult, and may therefore inhibit GABS in such a way as to modify the antigenicity and directly toxic effects. That the toxic products of GABS can find direct access from the pharynx to the heart region is demonstrated by a Russian study showing direct lymphatic pathways from the pharynx to the pericardial regions.

Whatever the exact pathogenesis, it is generally accepted that a child may develop ARF after 8-9 days of untreated pharyngitis with GABS. Because of the direct connection with pathogenesis, *vigorous documentation of antecedent GABS infection is critical before any consideration of ARF as a diagnosis is possible*. This may be in the form of throat culture in a medium with bacitracin [this selects GABS from other groups which are not sensitive to bacitracin] or in the form of serological data such as anti-streptolysin O antibody [ASO] titers. Remember that the normal ASO titer values in a given urban population may be as high as 250 Todd units. It is more convincing to observe a two tube dilution increase or decrease in ASO titer in temporal relation of ARF, than a borderline baseline value. GABS organisms elaborate many antigenic stimuli, including NADase [DPNase], DNAse, hyaluronidase, streptokinase, proteinase. Laboratory standards for anti-DNase B also exist. Newer slide agglutination tests such as Streptozyme [Wampole Laboratories] screen for many of the other antigenic responses, many of which persist much longer than ASO titer responses to GABS. The Streptozyme test screens for the following five antibodies: ASO, antistreptokinase, antihyaluronidase, antiDPNase, anti DNase. No *type specific* GABS is associated with ARF unlike acute glomerulonephritis which is associated with very type specific subgroups of GABS. In patients with previously documented ARF, proof of antecedent GABS upon suspected recurrent ARF is less necessary but should still be pursued.

Once GABS is confirmed, one has to evaluate the patient's entire clinical course in order to conclude that ARF is likely or not. Making a diagnosis of ARF has long term consequences in regard to the requirement and GABS prophylaxis and late cardiac sequelae. The Jones criteria are ordinarily divided into major and minor criteria. Minor manifestation, although not truly involved in a definitive diagnosis, often enable a more comprehensive evaluation of the patient. If one is able to identify one major criteria and two minor criteria or two major criteria, the diagnosis of ARF is most likely. The one exception to this involves the presentation of a child with *Sydenham's Chorea* between 5 and 15 years of age. This one finding alone enables the diagnosis of ARF. Importantly, this is usually such a late manifestation that serological evidence of antecedent GABS infection is not present. Why Dr. Jones included Sydenham's Chorea amongst the five major criteria instead of separating it, is still unclear to the author. Many clinicians are still confused when one makes the diagnosis of ARF solely upon the basis of Sydenham's Chorea, but this is a correct diagnosis and failure to make the diagnosis of ARF in this setting exposes the child to the possibility of recurrent ARF, possibly involving carditis. It is simple to conclude that a child presenting with Sydenham's Chorea must be placed on GABS prophylaxis. Other entities that may involve choreiform movements are idiopathic hypoparathyroidism, systemic Lupus Erythematosis, tumors, polycythemia.

Carditis: ARF may be associated with a pancarditis involving the myocardium, pericardium, and cardiac valves. Evidence of carditis involves detection of new, changing cardiac murmurs, specifically those of mitral and/or aortic insufficiency. Tricuspid and/or pulmonary insufficiency is possible but very rare. Acute phases of ARF involve inflammatory response and edema resulting in the above noted valvar insufficiencies, whereas late manifestation involve scarring and stenotic lesions predominantly of the mitral valve. Unfortunately even those children who have not had clinically active carditis during ARF are at risk of late development of mitral stenosis. Pericardial friction rubs may be included as evidence for carditis. Interestingly pericardial effusions associated with juvenile rheumatoid arthritis are much more severe than those associated with ARF. Overt CHF is possible if the acute mitral insufficiency is severe or a myocarditis is also present. Differentiation between cardiomegaly associated with pericardial effusion from that associated with CHF is possible with ECHO study.

Migrating Polyarthritis: Usually involving the large joints such as knees, ankles, elbows, and wrists, this major criterion classically involves swelling, erythema, marked tenderness and heat in the joint involved with subsidence of inflammation within two to three days at which time another large joint becomes inflamed. Rarely the hips are involved. It is very rare for the interphalangeal joints to be involved; this is much more common in juvenile rheumatoid arthritis. *If one uses migrating polyarthritis as a major criterion, one cannot use polyarthralgia as a minor criterion.*

Subcutaneous nodules: This could also be a relatively late manifestation of ARF. The lesion is a freely mobile painless subcutaneous lump dominantly found over the extensor surfaces of the joints such as elbows, knuckles, knees, and ankles. Do not fail to examine the paraspinal regions and the scalp for evidence of subcutaneous nodules as well.

Erythema Marginatum: This rash is a sharply marginated macular, pink rash occurring most frequently over the trunk and medial aspects of the upper arm and thigh. It may be very evanescent, and an old clinical trick involves observing the child after a warm bath which may bring out the rash more distinctly. Acute glomerulonephritis or drug reactions may produce this rash, which may also be idiopathic.

Minor Criteria: *Fever* usually ranges between 101-104° F and has diurnal variation. Within 24 hours after starting salicylate [ASA] therapy, temperature usually returns to normal and remains normal, dramatically. This response may indirectly further substantiate that the physician made a correct diagnosis of ARF, because so few illnesses with this degree of temperature elevation respond so well to salicylate therapy alone.

Arthralgia indicates joint pain without objective signs of inflammation. This may be migratory as well.

Laboratory criteria include: [1] Increased Erythrocyte sedimentation rate [ESR]. Note that in the face of significant CHF, ESR decreases toward 0 mm/Hour; [2] Increased C-reactive protein [CRP] is useful also. Many laboratories report CRP as 0 to 4+ with 0 to 2+ considered within normal ranges; [3] Leukocytosis; [4] PR interval prolongation toward first degree A-V block on the ECG. Clinically this may become associated with a decreased intensity of the first heart sound. It is not evidence of carditis, importantly.

Minor manifestations of ARF are of interest as supportive aids in diagnosis but are not used in isolation to confirm the diagnosis. These include severe abdominal pain, rapid sleeping pulse rate out of proportion to temperature elevation, anemia, malaise, epistaxis, precordial pain.

The following should be considered in the differential diagnosis of fever, polyarthritis and increased ESR: [1] rheumatoid arthritis, [2] systemic Lupus Erythematosis, [3] subacute bacterial endocarditis, [4] serum sickness, [5] sickle cell anemia, [6] tuberculosis, [7] undulent fever, [8] viral myocarditis, [9] leukemia, [10] septicemia especially meningococcemia, [11] atypical pneumonia or infection with PPLO organisms (17).

Therapy: Upon suspecting the diagnosis of ARF the physician should give an eradicating dose of penicillin for GABS, after appropriate throat cultures and even before results of serological tests. With carditis, or other severe forms of ARF it is most appropriate to use IM Benzathine Penicillin to eradicate GABS rather than oral regimens, because the recurrence rate of GABS is definitely less using Benzathine Penicillin. In children under 10 years 600,000-900,000 units is adequate; in children 10 year and older 900,000 to 1.2 million units is adequate for eradication. Oral regimens consist of 250,000 units of Penicillin G or V q 6 h for ten days. If using Penicillin G, attention to meals is necessary as this form should be taken on an empty stomach. With Penicillin allergy, erythromycin may be used orally given as 10 mg/kg/dose every six hours for 10 days, with a maximum dose of 200-250 mg/dose. Sulfonamides should not be used for eradication of GABS but are useful for prophylaxis.

Withhold salicylate therapy until a firm diagnosis is possible, because early salicylate therapy masks many of the important manifestation. Once the diagnosis is possible, salicylate [ASA] therapy is indicated unless there is significant carditis or the arthritis is extremely severe, in which case steroids are indicated. Mild carditis involving only mild mitral and/or aortic insufficiency usually responds well to ASA therapy alone. Furthermore there is no good data to suggest that steroid therapy avoids long term sequelae of carditis or better controls mild carditis. Doses of salicylates most useful are 3/4 to 1 Grain/lb/day [100-130 mg/kg/day] divided into 6 doses and given every 4 hours around the clock. For less severe illness the total daily dose may be divided into 4 doses given 6 hours apart, but this usually is inadequate to control more severe cases. Serum salicylate levels should be maintained around 20 mg% and serum samples should be obtained 2 hours after a given dose. ASA therapy continues until signs and symptoms resolve [usually 2-4 weeks]. If the episode of ARF is severe or prolonged, it is often beneficial to taper ASA therapy rather than suddenly stop therapy, to avoid rebound or recurrent symptoms.

In patients with severe ARF or with significant carditis one tends to use high dose steroid therapy such as Prednisone 60 mg/m^2/day or 2mg/kg/day divided into 2 to 4 doses per day. The author has used a combination of ASA and steroids in very severe cases of ARF. Furthermore it may be useful to add salicylate therapy as steroids are tapered, also to avoid rebound phenomenon. The timing of termination of steroid therapy in cases of carditis may be suggested by a return of CRP levels to normal, whereas ESR remains increased for longer periods of time.

If CHF develops, standard therapy with diuretics and digoxin may be used. Rarely mitral insufficiency is so severe as to require emergency valve replacement. Also rare but serious is the development of chronic rheumatic fever in a small group of children. When ARF was prevalent, many urban hospitals had wards filled only with chronic rheumatic fever patients. Pericardial effusion usually resolves with anti-inflammatory therapy; it rarely requires pericardiocentesis and rarely results in constrictive pericarditis.

Prophylactic regimens: Several options are available in long term prophylaxis against GABS. The most effective is monthly injection of 1.2 million units of Benzathine Penicillin. This would be the best alternative in patients with carditis upon first bout of ARF or with recurrent ARF.

Daily oral Penicillin G or V given as 200,000-250,000 BID is another alternative.

Sulfadiazine 0.5 Gm once daily in children under 50 lbs [25 kg] and 1.0 Gm once daily in children 50 lbs [25 kg] and over, is also useful. Note that this drug should not be used for primary eradication of GABS. Patients on this regimen should be monitored for leukopenia, fever, and rash.

In patients allergic to penicillin, erythromycin is useful in doses of 10 mg/kg/dose BID with a maximum dose of 200-250 mg BID.

A major question and point of confusion is when to stop GABS prophylaxis. The author suggests prophylaxis in patients with severe carditis or with a recurrent episode of ARF, for life. Most would consider stopping prophylaxis for milder form of ARF when the patient is 20 to 30 years old, provided any pharyngitis receives immediate attention thereafter.

Standard SBE prophylaxis is necessary in patients with cardiac sequelae such as mitral and/or aortic insufficiency. The author prefers that a patient not take an antibiotic at least one week before using SBE prophylaxis to allow a more normal flora to develop prior to SBE prophylaxis. Alternatively, if the patient is taking penicillin GABS prophylaxis, one could use erythromycin SBE prophylaxis.

Although the overall incidence of ARF in the United States has decreased markedly (18), there are still population centers within our country with high rates. In the Navajo population the annual rate was 12.4/100,000 population for all ages between 1962 and 1977. Rates as high as 96% occur in Hawaiin Samoans with a 50% incidence of associated carditis. It remains important for the younger physician to maintain an organized, sound approach to ARF in order to detect it and treat it appropriately.

Notes

1. Melish M: "Diagnosis and Management". Symposium III: Coronary Artery Problems: Mucocutanesous Lymph Node Syndrome. 28th Annual Meeting, American Academy of Pediatrics, Section on Cardiology, Washington D.C. 11/01/86.

2. Koren G, MacLeod SM: Difficulty in achieving therapeutic concentrations of salicylate in Kawasaki disease. *J Pediatrics* 105:991, 1984.

3. Takahashi M, Mason W: Letter to the editor. *Pediatrics* 77:617, 1986.

4. Furusho K, Nakano H, Shinomiya K, et al: High dose intravenous gammaglobulin for Kawasaki disease. *Lancet* 2:1055-1058, 1984.

5. Feigin RD, Barron KS: Treatment of Kawasaki syndrome [editorial comment]. *New Engl J Med* 315: 388-390, 1986.

6. Newburger J, et al: The treatment of Kawasaki syndrome with intravenous gammaglobulin. *New Engl J Med* 315: 341-347, 1986.

7. Kawasaki T: Symposium III: Coronary Artery Problems: Mucocutanesous Lymph Node Syndrome. 28th Annual Meeting, American Academy of Pediatrics, Section on Cardiology, Washington D.C. 11/01/86.

8. Burns JC, Glode MP, Clarke JW, Hathaway WE: Coagulopathy and platelet activation in Kawasaki syndrome: Identification of patients at high risk for development of coronary artery aneurysms. *J Pediatrics* 105:206,1984.

9. Koren G, Sasson L, Rose V,Rowe R: Kawasaki disease: Review of risk factors for coronary artery aneurysm. *J Pediatrics* 108:388-392, 1986.

10. Rowe RD. Kawasaki syndrome: Canadian update. *Can Med Assoc J* 132:237, 1985.

11. Fujiwara H, Chen C, Fujiwara T, Nishioka K, Kawai C, Hamashima Y: Clinicopathologic Study of Abnormal Q Waves in Kawasaki Disease [Mucocutaneous Lymph Node Syndrome]. *Am J Cardiology* 45: 797, 1980.

12. Gidding SS, et al: Mucocutaneous Lymph Node Syndrome [Kawasaki Disease]: Delayed Aortic and Mitral Insufficiency Secondary to Active Valvulitis. *J Am Coll Cardiol* 7:894-7, 1986.

13. Kawasaki T: Symposium III: Coronary Artery Problems: Mucocutanesous Lymph Node Syndrome. 28th Annual Meeting, American Academy of Pediatrics, Section on Cardiology, Washington D.C. 11/01/86.

14. Rauch A: "Epidemiology". Symposium III: Coronary Artery Problems: Mucocutanesous Lymph Node Syndrome. 28th Annual Meeting, American Academy of Pediatrics, Section on Cardiology, Washington D.C. 11/01/86.

15. Zabriskie JB: Rheumatic fever: the interplay between host, genetics, and microbe. *Circulation* 71:1077-1086, 1985.

16. Wannamaker LW: The Chain that Links the Heart to the Throat. *Circulation* 48:9-18, 1973.

17. Weinstein MP, Hall CB: Mycoplasma Pneumonia Infection Associated with Migratory Polyarthritis. *Am J Dis Child* 127: 125, 1974.

18. Gordis L: The virtual disappearance of rheumatic fever in the United States: lessons in the rise and fall of disease. *Circulation* 72:1155-162, 1985.

Chapter 9

Miscellaneous Cardiac Abnormalities

CARDIOMYOPATHY

Nomenclature and classification of cardiomyopathies have changed significantly over a short period of time as we gain better insight into this overlapping group of disorders. The most basic classification divides the group into primary and secondary. Goodwin provided a logical classification of primary cardiomyopathy, based upon function and anatomy: hypertrophic, congestive [or dilated], obliterative, restrictive (1).

Hypertrophic cardiomyopathy: The spectrum of this complex myocardial disorder is broad, but basically involves nondilated left ventricular hypertrophy with 90% of patients having disproportionate septal thickening compared with the left ventricular free wall. Etiology is genetically determined in 60% of patients according to an autosomal dominant transmission with variable penetrance. Male to female incidence ratio is 65:35. Interestingly, only 20% of relatives of an index case are affected because of the variability of transmission. Of those affected in a given family, only 33% have clinically significant forms of the disorder. The remainder have asymptomatic subclinical forms such as isolated asymmetric septal hypertrophy. "Malignant" hypertrophic cardiomyopathy would be suggested if a family had a history of several premature sudden cardiac deaths. It is the author's practice to suggest echocardiographic screening of family members relating to an index child, although some cardiologists limit such screening to families with poor histories only. In the other 40% of families where there is no genetic transmission, etiology is unknown and may include spontaneous genetic mutation. Secondary forms of hypertrophic cardiomyopathy occur with the following : pheochromocytoma, tuberous sclerosis, neurofibromatosis, lentiginosis, Friedrich ataxia, Turner Syndrome, Noonan Syndrome, hyperthyroidism. Pulmonary arterial banding and aortic valve replacement rarely become associated with subsequent hypertrophic cardiomyopathic pictures.

One of the most important associations with hypertrophic cardiomyopathy is significant dynamic subaortic obstruction largely relating to abnormal mitral valve motion [systolic anterior motion]. A useful physiological subclassification involves the degree of obstruction at rest or upon provocation such as isoproterenol infusion, amyl nitrite inhalation, or Valsalva maneuver: *obstructive*- resting systolic pressure difference of 30 mm Hg or more between the left ventricular sinus and aorta; *provocable*- resting systolic pressure difference of 30 mm Hg or more develops with provocation as noted above; *nonobstructive*- systolic pressure difference of less than 30 mm Hg at rest or with provocation. Difficulty in filling an abnormally hypertrophied left ventricle results in diastolic filling problems in some patients. Such a decrease in diastolic filling may occur in patients without subaortic systolic obstruction. Focusing upon the importance of the subaortic obstruction, earlier literature used the term idiopathic subaortic stenosis or IHSS to describe hypertrophic obstructive forms of cardiomyopathy, whereas recent papers refer to this entity as hypertrophic obstructive cardiomyopathy [HOCM].

Cardiac history in patients with hypertrophic cardiomyopathy usually begins with the detection of a non-specific murmur in childhood. Symptoms may be present at any age but usually affect patients between 20 and 40 years of age. The spectrum of symptoms includes infants presenting with congestive cardiac failure and no occurrence of symptoms until 60 to 70 years of age. Interestingly symptoms may occur in patients with or without subaortic obstruction and are not related to the severity of subaortic obstruction. Three-quarters of symptomatic patients suffer exertional dyspnea and/or excessive fatigue. Other symptoms include chest pain, dizziness, syncope, paroxysmal nocturnal dyspnea, and palpitations. Chest pain in not necessarily anginal in quality and its etiology remains uncertain apart from the logical notion that there is an imbalance between myocardial oxygen supply and demand, especially in face of subaortic obstruction. Arrhythmias such as atrial fibrillation are ominous and poorly tolerated. Fortunately such arrhythmias are unusual in patients less than 21 years old.

Physical findings in hypertrophic cardiomyopathy vary with the degree of subaortic obstruction and with the degree of diastolic filling compromise. With severe degrees of subaortic stenosis one is able to appreciate a very hyperdynamic apical impulse with the impression of a double or triple thrusting quality. The first heart sound is normal or accentuated. If accentuated, this finding may suggest associated pre-excitation conduction such as Wolff-Parkinson-White conduction. This association is fairly common. The second heart sound may be normal. With very severe subaortic obstruction there is a delay in the aortic component of the second heart sound, resulting in a narrowly split second sound. Rarely, the second heart sound is paradoxically split in the most severe forms of systolic obstruction. Fourth heart sounds may be present with marked decrease in ventricular compliance as well. Medium pitched, slightly harsh, relatively short systolic ejection murmurs are present between the mid to lower left sternal border and at the apex. Some have a somewhat innocent vibratory quality, but there are usually enough harsh overtones to suspect pathology. Some systolic murmurs are also longer, suggesting mitral insufficiency. With louder murmurs of dynamic subaortic obstruction, there is radiation toward the base and/or axilla. Occasionally we have heard typical high pitched short decrescendo, blowing diastolic murmurs of associated aortic insufficiency. Apical diastolic rumbles likely represent a decrease in left ventricular compliance resulting in difficulty with filling. There is seldom hepatomegaly, unless significant congestive cardiac failure exists. Pulses are characteristic with subaortic obstruction and are noted as prominent with a bisferens contour. This relates to the interruption of smooth left ventricular ejection as the dynamic subaortic obstruction develops during systole.

The ECG is variable, but abnormal in 90% of patients. Left ventricular hypertrophy with associated ST-T wave abnormalities are common. Left atrial abnormality, abnormal Q waves, and diminished or absent R waves in the lateral leads [pseudoinfarct pattern] are possible. There is no direct correlation between the degree of septal hypertrophy and the presence of abnormal Q waves. The 10% of patients with normal ECG patterns usually have no significant subaortic obstruction.

Radiographic findings are not diagnostic but demonstrate cardiomegaly in two thirds of patients. This cardiac enlargement reflects an increase in cardiac mass and left atrial size rather than left ventricular cavitary dilatation. Importantly, the presence or degree of cardiomegaly has no prognostic value.

We now consider echocardiographic findings quite typical in many cases, including asymmetrical septal hypertrophy with dynamic subaortic obstruction from systolic anterior motion of the mitral valve. Premature closure of the aortic valve is present with significant subaortic stenosis. In 10% of patients, the M-Mode echocardiogram is normal; however, cross-sectional [real-time] echocardiography usually demonstrates some abnormality consistent with the diagnosis. Real time echocardiographic patterns involve hypertrophy of the antero-lateral left ventricular free wall and ventricular septum in 55% of patients. In 20% of patients hypertrophy of the entire ventricular septum is present with normal left ventricular free wall dimensions. In 10% of patients hypertrophy is confined to the anterior ventricular septum. Patients with the most diffuse form of hypertrophy tend to have more functional limitation, resting subaortic obstruction, and left ventricular hypertrophy on the ECG.

Cardiac catheterization allows demonstration of the dynamic subaortic obstruction and in younger patients often allows demonstration of concomitant right ventricular subpulmonary obstruction. Provocation with intravenous isoproterenol infusion results in demonstration of systolic pressure drops as high as 50 to 100 mm Hg in patients with important dynamic subaortic obstruction. Generally drugs or maneuvers that decrease left ventricular afterload result in augmentation of subaortic obstruction, whereas increases in left ventricular afterload decrease subaortic obstruction. Drugs such as atropine, nitroglycerine, or amyl nitrite would worsen obstruction while phenylephrine, squatting, leg elevation or handgrip would lessen obstruction. Similarly, drugs or maneuvers that increase contractility increase subaortic obstruction, whereas a decrease in contractility would decrease obstruction. Isoproterenol and digitalis significantly increase obstruction, while beta blockade ameliorates obstruction. Decreases in left ventricular volume have similar adverse effects. Therefore, premature ventricular beats and Valsalva maneuvers worsen subaortic obstruction.

Natural history is very variable. One half of pediatric patients either succumb or experience deterioration. If heart failure develops within the first year of life, prognosis is very poor. Patients between 12 and 30 years old have the highest incidence of sudden death, which occurs in 35% of all patients with this pathology. Hypertrophic cardiomyopathy is a common cause of sudden death in the well conditioned athlete. If sudden death occurs in two or more family members the term "malignant" hypertrophic cardiomyopathy applies. Increased incidence of sudden death is associated with documentation of ventricular tachycardia on ECG monitoring. Syncope also appears to be associated with an increased risk, although this is not consistent. Importantly, there is no correlation between subaortic obstruction and sudden death, as one might expect. Finally one must consider the association with preexcitation conduction and potentially serious arrhythmias relating to sudden death. Summarily, 35% of patients with hypertrophic cardiomyopathy die suddenly, 23% remained stable, 25% deteriorate, and 17% appear to improve.

Therapy for this complex spectrum of hypertrophic cardiomyopathy usually involves attempts to decrease dynamic subaortic obstruction when present. Maneuvers that decrease afterload such as amyl nitrite should obviously be avoided. Therapy which increases contractility such as digitalis and beta agonists is essentially contraindicated. The classical form of therapy has involved administration of beta blocking agents in relatively high doses [e.g., 2-4 mg/Kg/day of propranolol]. In the patient with asthma, propranolol cannot be used. The author has has an excellent experience with use of a cardioselective beta blocking agent, acebutolol [Sectral], in an asthmatic teenager with severe hypertrophic obstructive cardiomyopathy, over a period of five years, with maintenance of very acceptable clinical stability. This patient also has Wolff-Parkinson-White [type B] syndrome. Newer therapeutic approaches involve calcium channel blocking agents such as verapamil, which often provide symptomatic relief. Unfortunately, neither propranolol nor verapamil appears to significantly prevent the feared event of sudden death in these patients, consistently. Amiodarone, a new antiarrhythmic agent, now appears to provide symptomatic improvement for these patients and may afford some protection against sudden death, but further studies are necessary to determine this. Amiodarone has many significant side effects, including thyroid dysfunction, pulmonary fibrosis, corneal deposits, and gray skin discoloration. Most of these side effects appear to be reversible upon discontinuation of this medication, which has an extremely long half-life.

Operative relief of severe subaortic obstruction [>50 mm Hg at rest or upon provocation] not responsive to medical therapy, may be beneficial using the Morrow procedure [transaortic ventricular septal myotomy-myomectomy] (2). Operative mortality is 5 to 10% and 9% of patients experience return of severe symptoms. There is an additional 7% late mortality from the disease process itself. Mitral valve replacement has been tried in order to relieve the subaortic obstruction but this procedure carries so many inherent risks of its own that it is seldom done now.

An important, reversible variant of hypertrophic cardiomyopathy involves the infant of a diabetic gestation who often demonstrates asymmetrical septal hypertrophy, possible systolic anterior motion of the mitral valve and cardiomegaly. They are at high risk as well for hypoglycemia and hypocalcemia, both of which are detrimental to neonatal cardiac performance. Ordinarily, this form of cardiomyopathy disappears within 6 to 9 months of age. Beta blockade is seldom necessary but if used, one should carefully monitor serum glucose, because propranolol therapy at this age may be associated with hypoglycemia.

Endocardial fibroelastosis [EFE]: This form of cardiomyopathy is either primary or secondary to congenital malformations of the heart such as aortic stenosis, aortic coarctation, mitral insufficiency or stenosis, aberrant origin of the left coronary artery from the pulmonary artery, patent ductus arteriosus, and hypoplastic left ventricle with aortic atresia. In the primary form, left ventricular involvement occurs with no associated cardiac abnormalities. This usually manifests in left ventricular dilatation but can result in a "contracted" left ventricle in 5% of patients. This severe disease occurs in 1/5000 live births and accounts for about 2-4% of all congenital cardiac diseases. The illness commonly affects infants and children between 2 months and 1 year of age with no gender difference and no racial differences. There has been some trend toward a decrease in incidence over the past several years. Etiology is undetermined but may involve antecedent viral infection with Coxsackie virus. Although usually sporadic, there are reports of some familial occurrences in which case genetic transmission may be operative. Patterns of hereditability include x-linked recessive, autosomal dominant with variable penetrance, and autosomal recessive.

Basic pathology involves marked left ventricular and left atrial enlargement with diffuse "milky-white" endocardial thickening, often most prominent in the subaortic region of the left ventricle. One half of patients demonstrate mitral or aortic valve involvement, resulting in functional insufficiency or stenosis.

History involves symptoms of progressive congestive cardiac failure in a previously healthy child. Presentation is within the first year in 80% of patients and within the first three months of age in 33%. Apart from classical signs and symptoms of congestive cardiac failure, infants may also present with fever, leukocytosis, skin rash or anemia. Frequent or recent upper respiratory infection is part of the history in 20% of children. Older children usually present less acutely with symptoms involving exertional dyspnea, orthopnea, easy fatigue, chest discomfort, abdominal pain, chronic dry cough, irritability, anorexia, vomiting and rarely diarrhea. Congestive failure may be so severe and so acute to cause presentation with cardiogenic shock and sudden death. Embolization of left ventricular or left atrial thrombi to the coronary or cerebral arteries may also cause sudden demise. Rarely EFE presents in adolescents or adults with one older patient surviving until 46 years of age.

Physical exam involves signs of congestive failure including easy diaphoresis, irritability, subcostal, intercostal, and/or suprasternal retraction, grunting, and a gray appearance or pallor. Heart and respiratory rates are increased. Systemic blood pressures are often low if the degree of congestive heart failure is considerable. The apical impulse is displaced laterally to the anterior or midaxillary line, consistent with a marked degree of cardiomegaly. Often the first and second heart sounds are diminished, having a "tick-tock" quality because of poor myocardial performance. Prominent third and/or fourth heart sounds are present. Murmurs are usually absent unless mitral insufficiency is present from the severe left ventricular dilatation. In this case, a soft, blowing systolic murmur may be present at the apex in 40% of patients at presentation and in as many as 50% or more of patients during later stages of the disease. Marked hepatomegaly is present in face of congestive cardiac failure.

Therapy involves vigorous stabilization of congestive cardiac failure with digitalis and diuretics. Once stable, the addition of afterload reduction with agents such as captopril or prazocin may also provide benefit, but are usually not necessary. The author prefers to add aldactone to any chronic diuretic regimen with furosemide or chlorothiazide in order to stabilize potassium balance and to inhibit aldosterone, which is demonstrably increased in most children with congestive cardiac failure.

The ECG demonstrates left ventricular hypertrophy in 70-95% of patients after the neonatal period. Lateral T wave inversion and prominent lateral q waves are frequent. With a chronic course resulting in pulmonary hypertension from left sided obstruction, biventricular hypertrophy may be present. Right ventricular hypertrophy is common in infants presenting with congestive cardiac failure in the first weeks of life, having the "contracted" form of EFE. Left, right or biatrial abnormalities are present in 35-60% of patients. One out of five patients have dysrhythmias or conduction blocks. Supraventricular arrhythmias, including atrial flutter and fibrillation are possible as well as ventricular dysrhythmias. Conduction blocks include complete left bundle branch block and may be as severe as complete heart block. Pre-excitation conduction such as Wolff-Parkinson-White syndrome also occurs in such patients.

Radiographic findings include marked cardiomegaly usually with dominant left ventricular enlargement. With dilatation of all cardiac chambers, globular shaped cardiac silhouettes are possible.

Echocardiographic findings generally include massive dilatation of the left ventricle and possibly left atrium. Fractional shortening is markedly decreased, consistent with very poor cardiac function. With better imaging capabilities it is possible to suspect the thickened "bright" endocardial surface in the left ventricle. Doppler flow evaluation would elaborate A-V valve insufficiencies.

If performed, cardiac catheterization would demonstrate marked increase in left ventricular end-diastolic pressures reflected in increased pulmonary arterial wedge pressures as well. In older children, pulmonary hypertension may reflect the decrease in left ventricular compliance and therefore difficulty filling the left ventricle.

Prognosis generally involves 33.3% complete recovery, 33.3% survival with persistent ECG abnormalities or clinical symptoms, and 33.3% demise with progressive congestive cardiac failure in spite of maximal therapy. Prompt recognition and initiation of vigorous anticongestive medication tends to promote better prognosis whereas neonatal presentation and recurrence of congestive cardiac failure while on therapy are poor prognostic signs.

Digitalis is usually continued for at least two to three years after initial therapy and only discontinued carefully if cardiac size and function appear to have returned to normal, in addition to ECG normalization. One-half of patients with a single episode of failure survive compared with 10% who have had three or more episodes. Rarely does an infant survive more than one month if presenting as a newborn. Ordinarily it is the newborn that presents with the contracted form of EFE, demonstrating pulmonary hypertension at this age secondary to markedly increased impedance to left ventricular filling. The left ventricle itself is normal or slightly small in size with more wall thickening but also with the diffuse endocardial thickening. Left atrial pressures are high, reflecting a poorly compliant left ventricle with high end diastolic pressure. ECG at this age shows right ventricular hypertrophy with associated ST-T wave abnormalities. Left or combined atrial abnormalities are also present.

In differentiating between hypertrophic cardiomyopathy [HM] and EFE in the infant, the echocardiogram usually demonstrates asymmetrical septal hypertrophy without left ventricular dilatation in HM. Poor systolic ventricular function associated with EFE is also helpful in the differential diagnosis. The rare anomalous left coronary arterial origin from the main pulmonary artery ordinarily demonstrates antero-lateral myocardial infarction on the ECG, but may be associated with secondary EFE and mitral insufficiency. Myocarditis may be the most difficult to differentiate but in only 10% of such cases is left ventricular hypertrophy present on ECG, whereas decreased QRS amplitudes are more common with myocarditis.

A relatively recent report indicates that systemic carnitine deficiency may present as familial EFE, and is potentially treatable. Therefore it seems appropriate to obtain serum carnitine levels [normal= 35-75 micro-mol/liter] and skeletal muscle carnitine levels [normal=3000-9000 nmol/g tissue] in children with familial cardiomyopathy of in any child with typical EFE (3).

<u>Idiopathic Congestive [Dilated] Cardiomyopathy [CC]</u>: Biventricular dilatation with increased myocardial mass but relatively normal wall thicknesses are characteristic of the pathological findings of CC. Absence of endocardial thickening differentiates CC from EFE while biventricular dilatation and absence of increased wall thicknesses differentiates CC from hypertrophic cardiomyopathy. As many as 75% of patients with CC have left ventricular thrombi as

a result of stasis from increased end-systolic ventricular volumes. Thrombi in the atrial appendages are also common. An obvious consequence of such thrombi is pulmonary or systemic embolization. Clinical course is relatively unknown because of the rarity of this entity and because patients with this form of cardiomyopathy were not necessarily separated from other forms in studies of prognosis. Presentation is similar to patients with EFE, with marked cardiomegaly and evidence for congestive cardiac failure. Physical findings are also similar including prominent third and/or fourth heart sounds. No murmurs or those murmurs of mitral insufficiency are present. ECG findings include non-specific ST-T wave abnormalities with atrial abnormalities, and may suggest a healed anterior wall infarction. Arrhythmias may be present as well.

CC may also present in infancy with rapid demise. The disease usually presents in older children and adolescents who may have a chronic course with eventual demise within five years. Treatment is similar to EFE therapy relating to aggressive use of anti-congestive medication. Although mostly sporadic, CC may be familial in which case it may appear to be genetically transmitted. A recent Mayo Clinic review of 24 patients [<1 month-18 years/ median 2 years] with CC indicates presentation with congestive cardiac failure in 92% of patients. Two-dimensional echocardiograms demonstrate left ventricular thrombus in 23% of patients studied [3/13]. Systemic arterial embolism occurred in 8% of patients upon follow-up. Survival at 1 year was 63% and at five years was 34%. In only 6/9 long term survivors, were there serial improvements of left ventricular function. Only one patient had severe mitral insufficiency. A recent viral syndrome was more common in survivors, but no clinical or laboratory variable consistently predicted outcome (4).

Miscellaneous cardiac muscle involvement: Glycogen storage disease, amyloidosis, myocardial iron deposition [e.g. in association with chronic anemias such as beta thalassemia], hypereosinophilic syndrome, and acromegaly are other causes of myocardial dysfunction. Barry J. Maron, M.D. has written an excellent review of the entire subject (5).

MYOCARDITIS

Pathological inflammation of the myocardium, pericardium, and endocardium may be caused by an enormous variety of organisms including viral, bacterial, atypical pneumonia agents, fungal, protozoal, Ricketsial, spirochetal, helminthic. The most common agents in children associated with myocarditis are viral, especially Coxsackie B, but including Coxsackie A, influenza, ECHO, mumps, and rubella. Presentation is ordinarily non-specific, including malaise, fever, lethargy and other viral symptoms. The most useful and potentially the most serious finding is the presence of any cardiac dysrhythmia or abnormality of conduction. ECG findings are very nonspecific as well and include nonspecific ST-T wave abnormalities with generalized flattening of T waves and ST segments. Ventricular hypertrophy is unusual. Any dysrhythmia is possible. Elevation of erythrocyte sedimentation rate and myocardial enzymes [LDH with isoenzymes and CPK with MB fractions] is possible.

Patient status ranges from nearly asymptomatic to cardiogenic shock with intractable ventricular or atrial dysrhythmias. Management relates to determination and therapy of the etiological agent when possible in addition to supportive therapy of the myocardial involvement. *Digitalis should be used cautiously in these patients because they appear sensitive to this medication and may develop digoxin related toxicity at standard doses of digoxin.* Newer recommendations of digitalization dose in Chapter 7, are likely low enough to avoid significant toxicity in patients with myocarditis but caution is nevertheless necessary. Stabilization of cardiac dysrhythmias and availability of pacemakers are necessary in many instances. The most controversial issue is whether one should use steroid therapy. In vitro studies suggest worsening of myocardial necrosis and increased viral replication with corticosteroids. It is likely safe to use steroids after the first ten days of involvement, but this is not completely known. Newer approaches involve use of immunosuppressive agents such as asathioprine, with promising results.

PANIC ATTACK SYNDROME

Although not newly described, one must consider a diagnosis of panic attack syndrome in a child with at least four of the following symptoms (6):

[1] Dyspnea

[2] Palpitations
[3] Chest pain or discomfort
[4] Choking or smothering sensations
[5] Dizziness, vertigo, or unsteady feeling
[6] Feelings of unreality
[7] Paresthesias [tingling of hands or feet]
[8] Hot and cold flashes
[9] Sweating
[10] Faintness
[11] Trembling or shaking
[12] Fear of dying, of "going crazy," or of doing something uncontrolled during an attack.

Other diagnostic criteria include the following:

[1] At least three such episodes occur within a three week period in circumstances other than marked physical exertion or a life-threatening situation. The attacks are not precipitated by exposure to a circumscribed phobic stimulus.
[2] The disorder is not due to a physical disorder or another mental disorder, such as major depression, somatization disorder, or schizophrenia.
[3] The disorder is not associated with agoraphobia.

The author has identified several children presenting for cardiac evaluation with panic attack syndrome. One responded very well to temporary [six month] propranolol therapy with no return of symptoms after further reassurance. The entity is often familial and likely involves a metabolic defect. Mitral valve prolapse occurs in as many as 30-50% of patients with panic attack syndrome.

Investigators at Mayo clinic suggest imipramine hydrochloride as a first step in therapy [25 mg BID]. If this does not control symptoms propranolol usually works well. If not, phenelzine may be tried followed by benzodiazepine. One author suggests that alprazolam may also be very beneficial, but *it should not be used in children* because of addiction potential and risk of severe withdrawal symptoms.

SYSTOLIC CLICKS

One of the most interesting and frustrating clinical findings relating to the cardiac exam is the detection of a systolic click. Only recently have pediatricians been able to recognize such sounds. which are important from the point of view that the majority of causes of systolic clicks require protection with SBE prophylaxis. A common cause of early systolic or ejection click is bicuspid aortic valve, which generally occurs in 6% of the entire population according to necropsy study. Although usually benign in childhood apart from possible mild to moderate associated aortic insufficiency, the older patient with isolated bicuspid aortic valve may develop stenosis. This connection remains to be proven further. Clinical findings in patients with bicuspid aortic valve include a distinct early systolic click located anywhere between the cardiac apex and aortic area at the upper right sternal border. Importantly such a click may actually be loudest at the midsternal edge, although usually present as well over the aortic area. With careful exam one might appreciate an almost subliminal, echoing, high pitched, decrescendo, blowing diastolic murmur also between the aortic area and apex, immediately after the aortic component of the second heart sound. With increasing degrees of aortic insufficiency, one is also able to appreciate a hyperdynamic apical impulse and prominent peripheral pulses with wide pulse pressure [systolic minus diastolic pressures]. The ECG is usually normal but would show LVH with severe aortic insufficiency. Echocardiography is usually diagnostic, although occasionally confusing. Most often there are three sinuses of Valsalva which are notably asymmetrical as are the aortic valve leaflets both on cross sectional exam and M-mode study. Diastolic fluttering of the mitral valve may indicate significant aortic insufficiency as would increased LV and aortic dimensions. Doppler evaluation is very sensitive in elaborating the presence and degree of aortic insufficiency. Naturally history is usually very benign with only a rare patient developing significant aortic insufficiency in childhood. Late occurrence of aortic stenosis is possible as already noted. No limitation of activity is necessary unless moderate or severe aortic insufficiency is present. SBE prophylaxis is very necessary.

Another interesting etiology for systolic clicks is a transient ventricular septal aneurysm upon spontaneous closure of a ventricular septal defect. Such a click is usually loudest at the mid left sternal border. Although almost always benign and most often transient, some VSD aneurysms can be large enough to obstruct the pulmonary outflow region, causing significant pulmonary stenosis, physiologically. Occasionally the aneurysm flips across the tricuspid valve resulting in a direct left ventricular to right atrial shunt if it is not completely closed, or causing tricuspid regurgitation. Importantly, such a child requires SBE prophylaxis even if the aneurysm is not complicated and even if the VSD has closed. Once there is no echocardiographic and/or clinical evidence for a residual aneurysm, the patient does not require SBE prophylaxis.

Any great vessel dilatation may cause a systolic click. A good example is aortic dilatation in patients with tetralogy of Fallot. In such patients a loud aortic ejection click is common. The degree of pulmonary stenosis is too severe to be associated with a click, for which reason the click likely originates from aortic dilatation resulting from the aorta carrying both the normal systemic cardiac output in addition to the right to left intracardiac shunt. Children with a large VSD may have dilatation of the pulmonary artery associated with the increased pressure and flow, and often have an associated systolic click in the pulmonary area of auscultation.

Mild to moderate aortic and pulmonary valve stenosis are other common causes from systolic ejection clicks. With aortic stenosis, the click is often maximal over the aortic area at the upper right sternal border and is constant, whereas with pulmonary stenosis the click is often maximal over the pulmonary area at the upper left sternal border and intermittent. All of these lesions require SBE prophylaxis.

An unusual entity not well described recently involves idiopathic dilatation of the main pulmonary artery, which also may result in a systolic click over the pulmonary region. This likely results from mild pulmonary stenosis early in childhood which resolves later, leaving only dilatation of the pulmonary artery. This entity is basically the only one associated with a systolic click that does not require SBE prophylaxis.

The most common cause for early and mid to late systolic clicks is mitral valve prolapse [MVP]. Occurring perhaps in as many as 8-16% of females and as many as 4-8% of males, this heterogeneous group of patients often presents a challenge in diagnosis and management. The classical form of mitral valve prolapse is associated with a mid systolic click or multiple clicks as well as a mid to late systolic murmur. In children it is more common to appreciate an early systolic click. Importantly the click need not be maximal directly at the apex, but is often present between the apex and lower left sternal border. Usually the click is loudest with the child sitting. The murmur is non-specific but usually has some regurgitant overtones. Associated innocent vibratory Still's murmurs may be present. A fascinating associated murmur is the systolic honk or whoop, which resembles the honk of a goose and may be loud enough for one to appreciate without the aid of a stethoscope (7,8). Associations apart from gender include thoracic skeletal abnormalities (9) [narrow thoracic antero-posterior diameter, straight back syndrome, pectus excavatum, and scoliosis], Von Willebrand Disease, Sickle Cell Disease, and slender habitus. Most patients with Marfan syndrome have mitral valve prolapse. It is also quite common to find mitral valve prolapse in patients with left ventricular volume overload from VSD or PDA or with left ventricular afterload problems such as hypertrophic obstructive cardiomyopathy or aortic coarctation. History often relates palpitations which are often ventricular in origin in children but may also be atrial in origin. The most serious association is prolonged QTc interval syndrome with possible syncope and sudden death from serious ventricular dysrhythmias. Panic attack syndrome may be associated with MVP, and autonomic imbalance may be present. Fortunately, the natural history of mitral valve prolapse in children is extremely good and there is no need to worry parents or children about the very rare instances of serious complications. Some children complain of non-anginal chest pain, which usually abates with reassurance and rarely requires therapy with beta blocking agents such as propranolol. Chest pains in children are generally not cardiac in origin but rather caused by musculoskeletal injury or inflammation, intercostal neuralgia, or esophageal spasm. The author finds that physicians often overlook esophageal spasm as a cause for chest pain in children and yet that it is quite common.

SBE prophylaxis is required for MVP especially with associated mitral insufficiency. Its use in the instance of isolated click is debatable but the author recommends SBE in such cases because of isolated reports in the literature describing several patients with SBE who had a systolic click only, in association with MVP. ECG findings are quite interesting and apart from the possibility of QTc interval prolongation, involve flattening or inversion of the inferior [Leads II,III,AVF] and/or lateral [Leads V5-6] T waves. The author has recognized that many children with mitral valve prolapse clinically, develop inverted or very flat T waves in Leads III and AVF of their ECG upon sitting, if such findings were not present in a reclining position. Unfortunately, some normal children may also demonstrate this findings although much less commonly. It is not certain whether such normal children with these changes have covert mitral valve prolapse, because echocardiograms have not yet been obtained in this group. The author believes that future research is necessary to define the rare patient with mitral valve prolapse who may develop significant complications as well as SBE. It is probable that future studies will enable a more logical recommendation of SBE prophylaxis in only a subset of the entire group with MVP. Doppler studies are important to assess the presence and degree of mitral insufficiency.

There has been some renewed interest in another fascinating and probably frequent cause of systolic clicks, tricuspid valve prolapse (10). Natural history and symptoms appear similar compared with MVP although this is not known with certainty because there is not yet enough experience with this entity in children. As an isolated phenomenon in the adult it is ordinarily associated with other severe cardiac disease or congenital malformation including dilated cardiomyopathy, systemic hypertension, mitral regurgitation due to chordal rupture, pulmonary hypertension, atrial septal defect, mitral stenosis, pericardial effusion, endocarditis and right ventricular trauma. The presence of tricuspid valve prolapse may explain the small group of children with systolic clicks consistent with mitral valve prolapse who have no echocardiographic evidence for MVP. The author has now found several children with tricuspid prolapse in lieu of or in addition to mitral prolapse when systolic clicks were not maximal at the apex, but rather at the lower left sternal border. Much more study is necessary to elaborate the implications of this entity in children. SBE prophylaxis is probably necessary although this is not known with certainty.

BACTERIAL ENDOCARDITIS

Eighty to ninety-five percent of all cases of bacterial endocarditis in children still involve either streptococci [viridans much more common than enterococci] and staphylococci [aureus more common than epidermidis]. Basic concepts involve bacteremia associated with a congenital cardiac malformation such as ventricular septal defect or aortic stenosis. Usually benign lesions such as mitral valve prolapse, transient ventricular septal aneurysms after spontaneous VSD closure, and bicuspid aortic valve may all be associated with bacterial endocarditis. Symptoms may be very subtle and therefore one must rely upon a high index of suspicion in any child with known cardiac defect that develops an unexplained prolonged febrile episode. The following table is useful in reviewing usual clinical and laboratory findings:

Table 9.1: Frequent Clinical and Laboratory Findings Associated with Bacterial Endocarditis (11)

CLINICAL FINDINGS:	FREQUENCY:
Fever	Very Common
New or changing heart murmur	Very Common
Myalgia, arthralgia, headache, malaise	Majority/ Very Common
Congestive Heart Failure	Infrequent/ Majority
Petechia	Majority
Embolic phenomena	Infrequent/ Majority
Splenomegaly	Infrequent/ Majority
Embolic pneumonia	Infrequent/ Majority
Osler nodes or Janeway lesions	Rare/ Infrequent

[Osler nodes are red painful intradermal nodes in the pads of the finger and toes]
[Janeway lesions are painless hemorrhagic spots on the palms and soles]
[Roth spots are retinal hemorrhages with central clearing and are also possible]

LABORATORY FINDINGS:	FREQUENCY:
Positive blood culture off antibiotics	Very Common
Positive acute phase reactants	Very Common
Anemia	Majority
Hematuria	Majority
Positive rheumatoid factor	Infrequent
Leukocytosis	Infrequent

The most important aspect of diagnosis and appropriate therapy is isolation of the causative agent by blood culture, if possible. Generally it is the total volume of blood that allows the greatest yield, and notions of higher yields with blood cultures during fever spikes appear inaccurate. Therapy of endocarditis associated with very penicillin sensitive streptococci [minimal inhibitory concentration of penicillin less than or equal to 0.2 micrograms/ml], three basic regimens result in very high cure rates with little recurrence: [1] 4 weeks intravenous aqueous penicillin G 150,00 units/kg/day administered continuously or in every six hour doses; [2] 4 weeks of intravenous penicillin G as above with 2-4 weeks of parenteral aminoglycoside [gentamycin 2.5 mg/kg/dose up to 80 mg intravenously every 8 hours or amikacin 7.5 mg/kg/dose up to 240 mg intravenously every 8 hours]; [3] 2 week combined intravenous penicillin G and intravenous aminoglycoside therapy. It must be emphasized that regimens such as two week therapy should be used only in the most sensitive group of organisms and in the most stable, least affected patients.

Antibiotic therapy must be individualized in patients having other less sensitive organisms, based upon culture and sensitivity results as well as the degree of cardiac involvement. In the most serious instances of marked destruction of an aortic or mitral valve associated with severe congestive heart failure, it is occasionally necessary to replace such a valve surgically, although this carries great risk of recurrent endocarditis.

Prevention of subacute bacterial endocarditis [SBE] involves dental, ENT, and G-U prophylaxis as recently revised by the American Heart and Dental Associations. Importantly no specific regimen works completely and it remains uncertain as to whether many mild lesions such as minimal mitral valve prolapse require SBE prophylaxis. The author takes the position that all children and adults with these mild lesions require SBE prophylaxis because there are case reports of SBE developing rarely in patients with isolated mitral valve prolapse and no associated mitral insufficiency. A recent study indicates that 5/14 patients aged 8-21 years had SBE associated with Haemophilus parainfluenza, suggesting possible better prophylaxis with ampicillin in lieu of penicillin G (12). Ampicillin is presently used often as SBE prophylaxis in England. The above noted study was retrospective, however, and the question of appropriate SBE prophylaxis remains unanswered, completely. The following are the revised recommendations for SBE prophylaxis (13):

<u>Dental and Upper Respiratory Tract Surgical Procedures</u> [patients with isolated secundum ASD, six months post PDA ligation, and 6 months post secundum ASD repair without prosthetic patch did not require prophylaxis; beware that

there is a high association between ASD and mitral valve prolapse, however].

Examples of procedures requiring SBE prophylaxis included all dental procedures associated with gingival bleeding [not simple orthodontic adjustments or shedding of decidual teeth]; tonsillectomy and/or adenoidectomy; surgery including biopsy involving respiratory mucosa; bronchoscopy; incision and drainage of infected tissue; genitourinary and gastrointestinal such as cystoscopy, prostatic surgery, urethral catheterization, urinary tract surgery, vaginal hysterectomy, gallbladder surgery, colonic surgery, esophageal dilatation, sclerotherapy of esophageal varices, colonoscopy, upper GI endoscopy with biopsy or proctosigmoidoscopic biopsy.

ANTIBIOTIC REGIMENS FOR DENTAL/ RESPIRATORY TRACT PROCEDURES:

Standard Regimen:

Penicillin V 2.0 G PO 1 hour before procedure and 1.0 G PO 6 hours later.

Children less than 60-70 lbs, should receive one half the above dose.

Patients unable to receive oral medication may receive 2 million Units aqueous Penicillin G IV or IM 30-60 minutes before a procedure and 1 million units 6 hours later IM or IV.

Children may receive 50,000 Units/Kg aqueous Penicillin G 30-60 minutes before a procedure and 25,000 Units/Kg Penicillin G 6 hours later IM or IV, with maximum doses as outlined for adults.

Special Regimens:

[1] Parenteral regimen for maximal protection in patients with prosthetic valves, for example: Ampicillin 1-2 G IM or IV plus Gentamycin 1.5 mg/Kg IM or IV 30 minutes before a procedure, followed by 1 G penicillin V PO 6 hours later or one repeat dose of the parenteral regimen 8 hours later.

Children may receive Ampicillin 50 mg/Kg per dose and gentamycin 2 mg/Kg/dose.

[2] Oral regimen for patients allergic to penicillin: Erythromycin 1 G 1 hour before procedure PO, then 500 mg 6 hours later PO.

Children may receive Erythromycin 20 mg/Kg initially, then 10 mg/kg 6 hours later PO, with maximum dose as outlined for the adult.

[3] Parenteral regimen for patients allergic to penicillin: Vancomycin 1 G IV slowly over 1 hour before procedure with no repeat dose.

Children may receive Vancomycin 20 mg/Kg IV slowly over one hour before a procedure, with a maximum of 1 G.

ANTIBIOTIC REGIMENS FOR GI/GU PROCEDURES:

Standard regimen: Ampicillin 2 G IM or IV plus gentamycin 1.5 mg/Kg IM or IV 30-60 minutes before procedure. A similar follow up dose may be given 8 hours later.

Children may receive Ampicillin 50 mg/Kg/dose IV or IM and gentamycin 2 mg/kg/dose IV or IM with a maximum Ampicillin dose of 2 G.

Special regimens:

[1] Oral regimen for minor or repetitive procedures in low risk patients: Amoxicillin 3 G PO 1 hour before a procedure and 1.5 G PO 6 hours later.

Children may receive Amoxicillin 50 mg/Kg/dose initially, then 25 mg/Kg/dose 6 hours later with a maximum dose as outlined for the adult.

[2] Parenteral regimen for patients allergic to penicillin: Vancomycin 1 G IV slowly over 1 hour before procedure. No repeat dose necessary.

Children may receive Vancomycin 20 mg/Kg/dose with a maximum of 1 G IV slowly over 1 hour before procedure. No repeat dose is necessary.

Notes

1. Goodwin JF, Oakley CM: The cardiomyopathies. *Br Heart J* 34:545,1972.

2. Morrow AG: Hypertrophic subaortic stenosis. Operative methods utilized to relieve left ventricular outflow obstruction. *J Thorac Cardiovasc Surg* 76: 423, 1978.

3. Tripp ME, Katcher ML, Peters HA, Gilbert EF, Arya S, Hodach RJ, Shug AL: Systemic Carnitine Deficiency Presenting As Familial Endocardial Fibroelastosis. *NEJM* 305: 385, 1981.

4. Taliercio CP, Seward JB, Driscoll, DJ, Fisher LD, Gersh BJ, Tajik AJ: Idiopathic Dilated Cardiomyopathy in the Young:Clinical Profile and Natural History. *JACC* 6: 1126, 1985.

5. Maron, BJ: Cardiomyopathies. In Adams FH, Emmanoulides GC (eds): *Heart Disease in Infants, Children, and Adolescents*, 3rd Edition. Baltimore, Williams & Wilkins, 1983, p 757.

6. Van Winter JT, Stickler GB: Panic Attack syndrome. *J Pediatrics* 105:661-665, 1984.

7. Felner JM, Harwood S, Mond H, Plauth W, Brinsfield D, Schlant RC: Systolic Honks in Young Children. *Am J Cardiol* 40:206,211, 1977.

8. Behar VS, Whales RE, McIntosh HD: The Ballooning Mitral Valve in Patients with the "Precordial Honk" or "Whoop". *Am J Cardiol* 20:789-795, 1967.

9. Salomon J, Shah PM, Heinle RA: Thoracic Skeletal Abnormalities in Idiopathic Mitral Valve Prolapse. *Am J Cardiol* 36:32-36, 1975.

10. Weinreich DJ, Burke JF, Bharati S, Lev M: Isolated Tricuspid Valve Prolapse. *JACC* 6:475-81, 1985.

11. Modified from Kaplan EL, Shulman ST: *Endocarditis.* In Adams FH, Emmanoulides GC (eds): *Heart Disease in Infants, Children, and Adolescents*, 3rd Edition. Baltimore, Williams & Wilkins, 1983, p 569.

12. Harris JP, et al: Infective Endocarditis in Pediatric Mitral Valve Prolapse: A Multicenter Review. AAP Abstract. *Am Heart J* 112:646, 1986.

13. Shulman ST, et al: Prevention of Bacterial Endocarditis. A Statement for Health Professionals by the Committee on Rheumatic Fever and Infective Endocarditis of the Council on Cardiovascular Disease in the Young. *Circulation* 70:1123A-1127A, 1984.

Chapter 10

Sudden Death: Prevention and Denouement

The sudden death of a child without premonition is always tragic. Whether such sudden deaths could be avoided if screening programs develop is controversial. Experience from Kobe, Japan, indicates that apart from cardiomyopathy, sudden death during or just after vigorous exercise might be avoided by parent questionnaire, and ECG screening combined with pediatric cardiology exam. Dr. Kunizo Baba from Kobe General Hospital reported at the Second World Congress of Pediatric Cardiology [New York, 1985], that since 1973, only two sudden cardiac deaths occurred in children during the screening program compared with an incidence of 42 sudden deaths in the rest of the Hyogo prefecture. Of 212,356 six year old children screened between 1973 and 1983, 893 had at least one criterion to prompt cardiac evaluation. Of those 893 children, 718 had organic heart disease with 175 having ECG abnormalities and with 84 who were considered at high risk of sudden death.

Reviewing the issue of sudden death in American athletes, one finds that in athletes younger than 35 years old, sudden death is predominantly due to cardiovascular disease with hypertrophic cardiomyopathy accounting for 48% of the events. Other important causes of death in young athletes include idiopathic LV hypertrophy [18%], congenital coronary arterial anomalies including left coronary artery arising from the right sinus of Valsalva, right coronary artery arising from the left sinus of Valsalva, single coronary artery [left absent], hypolplasia of the right and left circumflex coronary arteries, and origin of the left main, left anterior descending, or the right coronary artery from the pulmonary trunk [14%], coronary heart disease [10%], ruptured aorta associated with cystic medial necrosis [7%]. Unexplained deaths represent 3% of the group. Myocardial bridging or tunneling of a major coronary artery such as the left anterior descending is no longer considered an important cause or potential for sudden death, in that at least 20% of all hearts at necropsy have such findings. Very rare causes of sudden death include intussusception of a large ramus intermedius coronary artery branch of the left main coronary artery, aortic valve papilloma occlusion of a coronary ostium, myocarditis, mitral valve prolapse [presumably associated with a serious cardiac dysrhythmia such as associated with prolonged QTc interval syndrome], aortic stenosis, and sarcoidosis.

Patients older than 35 years of age usually die suddenly from coronary heart disease [80%], with the remainder of sudden deaths associated with hypertrophic cardiomyopathy, mitral valve prolapse, acquired valve disease, and unexplained events (1).

It is important to realize that the highly trained athlete usually manifests increased LV diastolic dimensions [9.8% above expected normal] and/or increased LV posterior wall thickness [18.9% above normal] and/or septal thickness [14.3% above normal]. Occasionally an athlete will even demonstrate asymmetrical thickening of the anterior basal septum mimicking nonobstructive hypertrophic cardiomyopathy. However, the majority have normal septal/free wall ratios of less than 1.3/1.0.

Effects of athletic training in children appear to differ from the adult cardiac response significantly in that a study of 77 competitive swimmers between 5 and 17 years old demonstrated increased septal, LV wall, RV wall and RV cavity dimensions, whereas only 30% demonstrated an increased LV diastolic dimension (2).

Because it is important to detect the athlete with hypertrophic cardiomyopathy and distinguish that individual from the athlete with expected increased LV and wall dimensions, Dr. Barry Maron proposes general guidelines for echocardiographic distinction in the adult athlete (3):

VARIABLE	ATHLETE HEART	NONOBSTRUCTIVE HYPERTROPHIC CARDIOMYOPATHY	"GRAY ZONE"
Ventricular septal thickness [mm]	<15	>15	13-15
Septal/free wall ratio	<1.3/1.0	>/= 1.3/1.0	1.2-1.4/1.0
LV end-diastolic dimension [mm]	Normal or increased	Normal or decreased	Normal
Ejection fraction	Normal	Normal or increased	Normal
Abnormal ECG	25-50%	about 90%	Normal or abnormal

PREVENTIVE PEDIATRIC CARDIOLOGY

Issues relating to primary prevention of coronary artery disease [CAD] in the pediatric patient are usually clouded by arguments insisting that no controlled data exists to demonstrate that lowering serum cholesterol levels in children will result in a lower mortality and morbidity from coronary artery disease in the adult, and by concerns about the safety of dietary alteration in the child relative to growth and development. Although these concerns are justifiable, newer controlled studies in adults definitively document lower risk of CAD with lower serum cholesterol levels. One must also appreciate data that the process of CAD begins in childhood. Several studies based upon pathology data have confirmed this point of view. A very recent study demonstrated no alteration in growth or sexual maturation in 73 children treated for heterozygous familial hypercholesterolemia using diet change and bile acid-binding resins. Therapy decreased serum cholesterol into a range associated with a reduction of coronary heart disease events in hypercholesterolemic men with similar cholesterol levels after therapy as well (4).

Other important factors relating to CAD include adverse effects of smoking, obesity, diabetes and hypertension.

Increased age and male gender also contribute to an increased risk. Certainly one must strive to control other factors if possible, but it now appears that an important, controllable factor is serum cholesterol level. Fasting plasma cholesterol is carried mostly in the low-density [beta] lipoprotein [LDL] with the remainder in the high-density [alpha] lipoprotein [HDL] and very low-density [-beta] lipoprotein [VLDL]. Higher levels of LDL increases risk for CAD whereas higher levels of HDL decreases risk for CAD. Triglycerides are dominantly carried in the VLDL fraction of plasma. Tables 10.1 and 10.2 below, summarize normal serum lipid values for children (5,6). For comparison, Table 10.3 lists newly suggested adult levels from a preventive point of view.

Table 10.1: Normal Plasma Lipid Values [5th and 95 %ile] in Male Children

AGE [YRS]	CHOLESTEROL [mg/dL] TOTAL		HDL		LDL		VLDL		TRIGLYCERIDE [mg/dL]	
	5th	95th	5th	95th	5th	95th	5th	95th	5th	95th
At birth		92	---	---	---	41	---	---		67
0-4	114	203	---	---	---	---	---	---	29	99
5-9	121	203	38	75	63	129	0	18	30	101
10-14	119	202	37	74	64	133	1	22	32	125
15-19	113	197	30	63	62	130	2	26	36	148

Table 10.2: Normal Plasma Lipid Values [5th and 95 %ile] in Female Children

AGE [YRS]	CHOLESTEROL [mg/dL] TOTAL		HDL		LDL		VLDL		TRIGLYCERIDE [mg/dL]	
	5th	95th	5th	95th	5th	95th	5th	95th	5th	95th
At birth		92	---	---	---	41	---	---		67
0-4	112	200	---	---	---	---	---	---	34	112
5-9	126	205	36	73	68	140	1	24	32	105
10-14	124	201	37	70	68	136	2	23	37	131
15-19	120	203	35	74	59	137	2	24	39	132

Table 10.3: Serum Cholesterol Level Relative to CAD Risk in Men and Women (7)

AGE [YRS]	SERUM CHOLESTEROL LEVEL [mg/dl] MODERATE RISK [>75TH %ile]	HIGH RISK [>95TH %ile]
20-29	>200	>220
30-39	>220	>240
40 +	>240	>260

During the conference establishing the adult risk levels in the above table, the following four recommendations pertained to children:

[1] "It is desirable to begin prevention in childhood because patterns of life-style are developed in childhood. The moderate-fat and moderate-cholesterol diets recommended for the population at large in this report should be suitable for all family members, including healthy children older than 2 years. For children, the diets should provide all nutrients in quantities adequate to growth and development and meet energy requirements. Excessive gain in weight should be avoided."

[2] "Children at 'high risk' should be identified primarily by carefully obtained family histories rather than routine screening. The history should include parents, grandparents, and all first-degree relatives. A family history of hypercholesterolemia or premature coronary heart disease should alert the physician to obtain at least two blood cholesterol determinations."

[3] "If the blood cholesterol level in such 'high-risk' children is above the 75th percentile [approximately 170 mg/dL for children aged 2 to 19 years], total and HDL [high-density lipoprotein] cholesterol measurements should be obtained. Those children with blood cholesterol levels between the 75th and 90th percentile [170-185 mg/dL] should be counselled regarding diet and other cardiovascular risk factors and then followed up at one-year intervals. Those with levels above the 90th percentile [>185 mg/dL] require special dietary instructions and close supervision with evaluation of other risk factors. A child with a blood cholesterol level above the 95th percentile [>200 mg/dL] on two occasions is in a special category and may have one of the hereditary hypercholesterolemias. Strict dietary intervention is indicated and will be sufficient for many

children. Nonresponders should be considered for treatment with a lipid-lowering agent, e.g., a bile-acid sequestrant [such as cholestyramine]. All family members should be screened."

[4] "Dietary management of children with elevated blood cholesterol levels should be part of a total management that includes regular exercise programs, maintenance of ideal weight, avoidance of excess salt, and avoidance of cigarette smoking."

In a recent, outstanding commentary relating to this entire problem, Dr. Peter O. Kwiterovich, Jr., provides a synthesis of prudent dietary recommendations for healthy children older than 2 years, consistent with guidelines of the Nutrition Committee of the American Heart Association, the Senate Select Committee on Nutrition, and the above noted National Institutes of Health Consensus Development Statement (8).

Recommendation [1]: Nutritionally adequate diet consisting of a variety of foods.
Practical Implication [1]: Satisfies recommended dietary allowances of the Food and Nutrition Board of the National Research Council for protein, vitamins and minerals.

Recommendation [2]: Caloric intake based upon growth rate and activity level.
Practical Implication [2]: Maintain growth curve and weight appropriate for height.

Recommendation [3]: Decrease total fat intake approximately to 30% of calories and saturated fat to 10% of calories.
Practical Implication [3]: Emphasize consumption of lean meat, fish, and poultry and decrease use of fatty meats; substitute vitamin D-fortified skim milk or low-fat milk for whole milk; broil or bake rather than fry foods.

Recommendation [4]: Moderate use of polyunsaturated fats [to no more than 10% of calories].
Practical Implication [4]: Use soft margarine rather than solid margarine or butter; use of vegetable oils such as safflower or corn oil rather than lard for cooking or salads.

Recommendation [5]: Lower cholesterol intake to <300mg/day.
Practical Implication: [5] Limit eggs to 2-3/week; practical implications 3 and 4 above.

Recommendation [6]: Maintain protein at about 15-20% of calories.
Practical Implication [6]: Protein of both animal and vegetable sources will provide all essential amino acids.

Recommendation [7]: Increase percent of calories from carbohydrates from about 50-55%, derived primarily from complex carbohydrates, and emphasize increase in fiber.
Practical implication [7]: Increase consumption of whole grain or enriched breads, whole grain, enriched and fortified cereals; increase consumption of fruits and vegetables; decrease consumption of desserts, snack foods, candy bars, sweets.

Serum cholesterol and triglyceride levels should be measured after a 12-16 hour fast at a time when diet is relatively stable. *First degree men less than 50 years of age or women less than 60 years of age with a history of myocardial infarction are strong indications that a familial hyperlipidemia may exist and children whose families have such histories should be screened, as should those with a first degree relative with known hyperlipidemia.*

Table 10.4 summarizes the forms of hyperlipidemia according to original Fredrickson classifications:

Table 10.4: Fredrickson Classification of Hyperlipidemia (9)

TYPE	ELEVATED LIPID	ELEVATED LIPOPROTEIN	CHILDHOOD PREVALENCE
I	Triglyceride	Chylomicrons	Rare
IIa	Cholesterol	LDL	Common
IIb	Cholesterol Triglyceride	LDL VLDL	Uncommon
III	Cholesterol Triglyceride	Beta VLDL [Cholesterol-rich VLDL remnant]	Very Rare
IV	Triglyceride	VLDL	Uncommon
V	Triglyceride Cholesterol	Chylomicrons VLDL	Very rare

An excellent recent synopsis for treatment of childhood hyperlipidemia begins by outlining recommendations that are suggested as useful for all pediatric patients, including smoking prevention, repetitive aerobic physical activity, avoidance of excess calories, and avoidance of alcohol. The objectives for the general pediatric population would be maintenance of ideal weight for height and of cardiovascular fitness (10). Adult recommendations for effective exercise to maintain cardiovascular fitness suggest that an exercise must be: [1] intense enough to increase heart and respiratory rates more than 60% of those expected with maximum work intensity according to age and gender, [2] maintained for at least 30 minutes, and [3] performed at least 3 times weekly or every other day. The best forms of exercise to achieve these goals include jogging, rowing, stationary cycling, swimming laps, running in place, jumping rope and cross country skiing. Alternative exercises that usually require more than 30 minutes to achieve appropriate increases in heart and respiratory rates, include bicycling, racquetball, soccer, squash, singles tennis, and walking. Activities that least contribute to cardiovascular conditioning include baseball, bowling, football, golf, softball and volleyball (11).

As noted in Chapter 1, other cardiovascular problems that may cluster within a family include hypertension, stroke, dysrhythmias, hypertrophic cardiomyopathy, mitral valve prolapse, and rarely some forms of congenital heart defects such as tetralogy of Fallot, ASD, aortic coarctation.

Regarding blood pressure, for participation in strenuous activities or organized athletic activities, the following are broad guidelines of upper normal blood pressure limits in children:

AGE [YRS]	BLOOD PRESSURE [mm Hg]
<6	120/70
6-9	130/75
10-13	135/80
14-17	140/85

For adults, the following guidelines exist:

Classification	Diastolic Pressure [mm Hg]
Normal	<85
High Normal	85-89
Mild Hypertension	90-104
Moderate Hypertension	105-114
Severe Hypertension	>115
	Systolic Pressure [mm Hg] when diastolic <90 mm Hg
Normal	<140
Borderline isolated systolic hypertension	150-159
Isolated systolic hypertension	>160

Early detection of hypertension is important and may require cardiovascular stress testing to elaborate the patient's response to exercise. The author recommends that every family reasonably limit their salt intake, especially those with histories of hypertension.

Activity and work recommendations for children with increased risk factors or various congenital cardiac defects now exist. It is important to use these guidelines only as a first step in final recommendations, which must reflect each individual's special circumstances. The recommendation that each child with mild mitral valve prolapse undergo exercise ECG prior to participation in competetive sport activities may be excessive in spite of the well known association between mitral valve prolapse and serious cardiac dysrhythmias, including those associated with prolonged QTc interval. The prevelance of mitral and now tricupsid valve prolapse appears to be too great to make such a recommendation in every child with mitral or tricuspid valve prolapse. Definitions of Recreational Activity Levels are as follows:

Category I: No Restiction including endurance training, interscholastic athletic competition, and contact sports.

Category II: Moderate Exercise including regular physical education classes, tennis, and baseball.

Category III: Light Exercies including nonstrenusous team games, recreational swimming, jogging, cycling, and golf.

Category IV: Moderate Limitation including school attendance, but no physical education class participation.

Category V: Extreme Limitation with homebound or wheelchair activities only.

Table 10.5 below summarizes definitions of occupational activity.

Table 10.5: Definitions of Occupational Activities

Category	I	II	III	IV	V
WORK	Very Heavy	Heavy	Medium	Light	Sedentary
Peak Load [cal/min]	7.6+	7.6+	5-7.5	2.6-4.9	2.5 or less
May Lift Objects [lbs]	100+	100	50	20	20
Frequent Lifting and/or carrying of objects [lbs]	50+	50	25	10	see A,below

A: Occasional lifting and or carrying of objects such as dockets, ledgers or small tools.

Using above definitions for both activity and work categories the following listing is a synopsis of recommendations rearranged according to activity and work groups.

Patients under group I Recreational and group I Occupational Activity include those with:

1. ASD, PDA, VSD regardless of surgery but with no pulmonary vscular obstructive disease [PVOD]
2. Post operative aortic coarctation with normal blood pressure*
3. Asymptomatic, mild mitral valve prolapse
4. Mild pulmonary stenosis, regardless of surgery
5. Isolated premature atrial beats
6. Isolated premature ventricular beats with otherwise normal heart
7. Wolff-Parkinson-White Syndrome

Patients under group I Recreational and group II Occupational Activity include those with:

1. Mild aortic or mitral insufficiency with normal heart size
2. Mild aortic stenosis regardless of surgery
3. Postoperative tetralogy of Fallot with RV systolic pressure less than 50 mm Hg*
4. Supraventricular tachycardia
5. Mild hypertension

Patients under group II Recreational and group II Occupational Activity include those with:

1. Complete heart block
2. Permanent artificial pacemaker
3. Ventricular tachycardia with otherwise normal heart

Patients under group II Recreational and group III Occupational Activity include those with:

1. Mild, asymptomatic mitral stenosis with normal heart size
2. Other major surgically corrected congenital cardiac defects such as complete transposition, and tricuspid atresia. Because this group is very heterogeneous, evaluate each patient separately for final individual recommendations.

Patients under group III Recreational and group III Occupational Activity include those with:

1. Moderate aortic insufficiency
2. Moderate aortic stenosis regardless of surgery
3. ASD, PDA, VSD with mild to moderate PVOD, regardless of surgery
4. Aortic coarctation with systemic hypertension regardless of surgery
5. Moderate to severe isolated systemic hypertension
6. Moderate pulmonary stenosis regardless of surgery
7. Postoperative tetralogy of Fallot with RV systolic pressure greater than 49 mm Hg or with marked cardiomegaly
8. Premature ventricular beats with congenital or acquired heart disease, regardless of surgery

Patients under group III Recreational and group IV Occupational Activity include those with:

1. Hypertroohic cardiomyopathy
2. Idiopathic pulmonary hypertension with pulmonary arterial systolic pressure less than one-half systemic systolic pressure
3. Other major unoperated or palliated congenital defects such as tricuspid or pulmonary atresia, or Ebstein anomaly. Because this group is very heterogeneous, evaluate each patient separately for final individual recommendations

Patients under group IV Recreational and group IV Occupational Activity include those with:

1. Severe aortic insufficiency
2. Severe aortic stenosis regardless of surgery
3. ASD, PDA, VSD with moderate to severe PVOD
4. Severe pulmonary stenosis regardless of surgery
5. Ventricular tachycardia with congenital or acouired heart disease regardless of operation

Patients under group IV Recreational and group V Occupational Activity include those with:

1. Congestive of dilated cardiomyopathy
2. Severe mitral insufficiency or stenosis with marked cardiomegaly and/or atrial fibrillation
3. Chronic, stable myocarditis over 3 month's duration
4. Idiopathic pulmonary hypertension with pulmonary arterial systolic pressure greater than one-half systemic systolic pressure

Patients under group V Recreational and group V Occupational Activity include those with:

1. Active myocarditis

Exercise testing is suggested for patients with aortic coarctation, mild mitral valve prolapse, and postoperative tetralogy of Fallot where RV systolic pressure is less then 50 mm Hg, prior to participation in competitive athletics (12).

DENOUEMENT

In no manual for house officers does one find a word of support toward becoming a mature, caring, sensitive, productive future physician. The author teaches third and fourth year medical students as well of Pediatric and other House Officers and Fellows. Often the author finds it necessary to digress from discussions of Pediatric Cardiology to remind physicians in training that *in order to convey a sense of well being to their future patients, they themselves must have such a sense of well-being.* The physician no less than any human being must be certain to establish correct priorities and secure enough time for relaxation, for reading, for friends and for family. If possible, the physician should try to practice preventive medicine in his or her own family, including regular exercise.

Patients require a sense of well being when seeking help for pain or illness. The physician must maintain an attitude that will convey such a sense of well being under the most adverse of circumstances. The author is not implying that the physician should provide false hopes and not convey important information that may be distressful, but is rather trying to convey that the physician can do so in a gentle, reassuring manner sparked with hope and a sense of well being. Involve the patient in their own recovery and have them take responsibility for getting well along with you. One of my cherished authors is Norman Cousins who knows first hand how important these concepts can be to a patient. Having survived ankylosing spondylitis and a myocardial infarction, Norman Cousins continued to maintain a positive approach to life with a sense of humor and joy of life. Each step of the way he made suggestions of alternate therapy with his physicians and took an active role in his own recovery. He found the usual hospital surroundings abhorrent and lacking in humanism. Every physician, young and old, should read his two books *Anatomy of an Illness As Perceived by the Patient* (13) and *The Healing Heart* (14).

We have far to go before we achieve a completely humanistic approach to medicine, but in the author's opinion, the only way to reverse the negative public opinion directed toward physicians is to return to a close patient-physician relationship in a humanistic setting. So often do patients wait for hours before seeing a physician, even though having an appointment. So often do patients and families leave a physician's office with a confused and axious expression. Medicine has made exciting, important advances during this last decade, including non-surgical approaches to relief of coronary artery disease, non-surgical relief of congenital pulmonary and aortic stenosis, and pharmacological maintenance or closure of a patent ductus arteriosus. What physicians in training need now are more role models for the actual practice of medicine which is no less an art today than it was centuries ago. It is unfortunately too common to observe insensitive, rude, and thoughtless behavior in many physicians. One must realize how strong an impact a physician's words may have upon patients and others. One must think carefully about ways to alleviate fear, ways to alleviate sorrow, and ways to alleviate anxiety.

With these thoughts in mind, the author wishes future and practicing physicians good health, peace of mind, and the ability to comfort their patients.

Notes

1. Maron BJ, Epstein SE, Roberts WC: Causes of Sudden Death in Competitive Athletes. *JACC* 7:204-214, 1986.

2. Allen HD, Goldberg SJ, Sahn DJ, Schy N, Wojcik R: A quantitative echocardiographic study of champion childhood swimmers. *Circulation* 55:142-145, 1977.

3. Maron BJ: Structural Features of the Athlete Heart as Defined by Echocardiography. *JACC* 7:190-203, 1986.

4. Glueck CJ, Mellies MJ, Dine M, Perry T, Paskarzewski P: Safety and Efficacy of Long-Term Diet and Diet Plus Bile Acid-Binding Resin Cholesterol Lowering Therapy in 73 Children Heterozygous for Familial Hypercholesterolemia. *Pediatrics* 78:338-348, 1986.

5. Modified from *Lipid Research Clinics Population Studies Data Book, Vol I: The Prevalence Study*, US Department of Health and Human Services, National Institutes of Health publication No 80-1527. Government Printing Office, July, 1980.

6. Weidman W, Kwiterovich P Jr, eds., et al: Diagnosis and Treatment of Primary Hyperlipidemia in Childhood. A Joint Statement for Physicians by the Committee on Atherosclerosis and Hypertension in Childhood of the Council of Cardiovascular Disease in the Young and the Nutrition Committee, American Heart Association. *Circulation* 74:1181A-1188A, 1986 [November].

7. National Institutes of Health, Consensus Development Conference Statement. Lowering blood cholesterol to prevent heart disease. *JAMA* 253:2080-2095, 1985.

8. Kwiterovich PO Jr: Biochemical, Clinical, Epidemiologic, Genetic, and Pathologic Data in the Pediatric Age Group Relevant to the Cholesterol Hypothesis. *Pediatrics* 78:349-362, 1986.

9. Weidman W, Kwiterovich P Jr, eds., et al: Diagnosis and Treatment of Primary Hyperlipidemia in Childhood. A Joint Statement for Physicians by the Cimmittee on Atherosclerosis and Hypertension in Childhood of the Council of Cardiovascular Disease in the Young and the Nutrition Committee, American Heart Association. *Circulation* 74:1183A, 1986 [November].

10 Ibid: p 1186A.

11. Riopel DA, chairman, et al: Coronary Risk Factor Modification in Children: Exercise. A statement for Physicians by the Committee on Atherosclerosis and Hypertension in Childhood of the Council on Cardiovascular Disease in the Young, American Heart Association. *Circulation* 74:1189A-1191A, 1986 [November].

12. Gutgesell HP, Chairman, et al: Recreational and Occupational Recommendations for Young Patients with Heart Disease. A Statement for Physicians by the Committee on Congenital Cardiac Defects of the Council on Cardiovascular Diasease in the Young, American Heart Association. *Circulation* 74: 1195A-1198A, 1986 [November].

13. Cousins N: *Anatomy of an Illness As Perceived by the Patient:Reflections on Healing and Regeneration*. New York, WW Norton and Company, Inc, 1979.

14. Cousins N: *The Healing Heart*. Boston, G K Hall, 1984.

Index